MR Imaging of the Knee

Editor

MK JESSE

MAGNETIC RESONANCE IMAGING CLINICS OF NORTH AMERICA

www.mri.theclinics.com

Consulting Editors
SURESH K. MUKHERJI
LYNNE S. STEINBACH

May 2022 • Volume 30 • Number 2

ELSEVIER

1600 John F. Kennedy Boulevard • Suite 1800 • Philadelphia, Pennsylvania, 19103-2899

http://www.mri.theclinics.com

MRI CLINICS OF NORTH AMERICA Volume 30, Number 2
May 2022 ISSN 1064-9689, ISBN 13: 978-0-323-81385-3

Editor: John Vassallo (j.vassallo@elsevier.com)
Developmental Editor: Arlene Campos

Magnetic Resonance Imaging Clinics of North America (ISSN 1064-9689) is published quarterly by Elsevier Inc., 360 Park Avenue South, New York, NY 10010-1710. Months of issue are February, May, August, and November. Business and Editorial Offices: 1600 John F. Kennedy Blvd., Ste. 1800, Philadelphia, PA 19103-2899. Customer Service Office: 3251 Riverport Lane, Maryland Heights, MO 63043. Periodicals postage paid at New York, NY and additional mailing offices. Subscription prices are $408.00 per year (domestic individuals), $1053.00 per year (domestic institutions), $100.00 per year (domestic students/residents), $455.00 per year (Canadian individuals), $1069.00 per year (Canadian institutions), $573.00 per year (international individuals), $1069.00 per year (international institutions), $100.00 per year (Canadian students/residents), and $275.00 per year (international students/residents). International air speed delivery is included in all *Clinics* subscription prices. All prices are subject to change without notice. **POSTMASTER:** Send address changes to *Magnetic Resonance Imaging Clinics*, Elsevier Health Sciences Division, Subscription Customer Service, 3251 Riverport Lane, Maryland Heights, MO 63043. Customer Service (orders, claims, online, change of address): Elsevier Health Sciences Division, Subscription **Customer Service, 3251 Riverport Lane, Maryland Heights, MO 63043. Tel:1-800-654-2452 (U.S. and Canada); 314-447-8871 (outside U.S. and Canada). Fax: 314-447-8029. E-mail: journalscustomerservice-usa@elsevier.com (for print support); journalsonlinesupport-usa@elsevier.com (for online support).**

Reprints. For copies of 100 or more of articles in this publication, please contact the Commercial Reprints Department, Elsevier Inc., 360 Park Avenue South, New York, NY 10010-1710. Tel.: 212-633-3874; Fax: 212-633-3820; E-mail: reprints@elsevier.com.

Magnetic Resonance Imaging Clinics of North America is covered in the *RSNA Index of Imaging Literature, MEDLINE/PubMed (Index Medicus),* and *EMBASE/Excerpta Medica.*

Contributors

CONSULTING EDITORS

SURESH K. MUKHERJI, MD, MBA, FACR
Clinical Professor of Radiology and Radiation
Oncology, University of Illinois, Peoria, Illinois,
USA; Robert Wood Johnson Medical School,
Rutgers University, New Brunswick, New
Jersey, USA; Faculty, Otolaryngology Head
Neck Surgery, Michigan State University,
Farmington Hills, Michigan, USA; National
Director of Head and Neck Radiology, ProScan
Imaging, Carmel, Indiana, USA

LYNNE S. STEINBACH, MD, FACR
Emeritus Professor of Radiology on Full Recall,
Department of Radiology and Biomedical
Imaging, University of California, San
Francisco, San Francisco, California, USA

EDITOR

MK JESSE, MD
Associate Professor of Radiology, Assistant
Professor of Orthopedics, Director of
Musculoskeletal Intervention, University of
Colorado Anschutz Medical Campus,
University of Colorado Hospital, Anschutz
Outpatient Pavilion, Department of Radiology,
Aurora, Colorado, USA

AUTHORS

ERIN ALAIA, MD
Department of Radiology, NYU
Langone Health, New York, New York,
USA

HAMZA ALIZAI, MD
Department of Radiology, Scottish Rite for
Children, Dallas, Texas, USA

HAILEY ALLEN, MD
Department of Radiology and Imaging
Sciences, University of Utah School
of Medicine, Salt Lake City, Utah,
USA

CONNIE Y. CHANG, MD
Division of Musculoskeletal Imaging and
Intervention, Department of Radiology,
Massachusetts General Hospital, Boston,
Massachusetts, USA

CEYLAN COLAK, MD
Department of Radiology, Imaging Institute,
Cleveland Clinic, Cleveland, Ohio,
USA

KIRKLAND W. DAVIS, MD, FACR
University of Wisconsin-Madison School of
Medicine and Public Health, Madison,
Wisconsin, USA

SONJA FIERSTRA, MD
Joint Department of Medical Imaging,
University Health Network, Mount Sinai
Hospital and Women's College Hospital,
Toronto, Ontario, Canada

DONALD FLEMMING, MD
Professor of Radiology and Orthopaedics,
Penn State Health Milton S. Hershey Medical
Center, Hershey, Pennsylvania, USA

KARA G. GILL, MD
University of Wisconsin-Madison School of
Medicine and Public Health, Madison,
Wisconsin, USA

SOTERIOS GYFTOPOULOS, MD, MBA, MSc
Departments of Radiology and Orthopedic
Surgery, NYU Langone Health, New York,
New York, USA

COREY K. HO, MD
Assistant Professor, Department of Radiology,
University of Colorado School of Medicine,
Aurora, Colorado, USA

WILLIAM W. KESLER, MD
Clinical Fellow, Diagnostic Radiology, Penn
State Health Milton S. Hershey Medical Center,
Hershey, Pennsylvania, USA

IMAN KHODARAHMI, MD, MSc, PhD
Department of Radiology, NYU Langone
Health, New York, New York, USA

ALEXANDER N. MERKLE, MD
Assistant Professor, Department of Radiology,
University of Colorado School of Medicine,
Aurora, Colorado, USA

MEGAN K. MILLS, MD
Department of Radiology and Imaging
Sciences, University of Utah School of
Medicine, Salt Lake City, Utah, USA

LANE MINER, DO
Clinical Instructor of Radiology, Penn State
Health Milton S. Hershey Medical Center,
Hershey, Pennsylvania, USA

WILLIAM B. MORRISON, MD, FACR
Department of Radiology, Thomas Jefferson
University Hospital, Philadelphia,
Pennsylvania, USA

MINI N. PATHRIA, MD
Professor of Clinical Radiology, Department of
Radiology, UCSD Health System, University of
California, HCOP MRI, San Diego, California,
USA

ADAM RUDD, MD
Department of Radiology, UCSD Health
System, University of California, HCOP MRI,
San Diego, California, USA

COLIN D. STRICKLAND, MD
Associate Professor, Department of Radiology,
University of Colorado School of Medicine,
Aurora, Colorado, USA

NAVEEN SUBHAS, MD, MPH
Department of Radiology, Imaging Institute,
Cleveland Clinic, Cleveland, Ohio,
USA

LUKAS M. TRUNZ, MD
Department of Radiology, Thomas Jefferson
University Hospital, Philadelphia,
Pennsylvania, USA

JOAO R.T. VICENTINI, MD
Division of Musculoskeletal Imaging and
Intervention, Department of Radiology,
Massachusetts General Hospital, Boston,
Massachusetts, USA

ARMANDO F. VIDAL, MD
The Steadman Clinic and Steadman
Philippon Research Institute, Vail, Colorado,
USA

CARISSA M. WHITE, MD
Assistant Professor of Radiology, Penn State
Health Milton S. Hershey Medical Center,
Hershey, Pennsylvania, USA

LAWRENCE M. WHITE, MD, FRCPC
Joint Department of Medical Imaging,
University Health Network, Mount Sinai
Hospital and Women's College Hospital,
Department of Medical Imaging, Temerty
Faculty of Medicine, University of Toronto,
Toronto, Ontario, Canada

FANGBAI WU, MD
Department of Radiology, Imaging Institute,
Cleveland Clinic, Cleveland, Ohio,
USA

Contents

whereas masses affecting multiple articulations are typically caused by underlying inflammatory arthritides, metabolic abnormalities, or systemic deposition disorders. This article focuses on those masses that present in a monoarticular fashion, emphasizing the lesions that most commonly affect the knee joint. MR imaging is the modality of choice for evaluation of knee masses, allowing specific diagnosis in most cases.

Sonja Fierstra and Lawrence M. White

Meniscal tears are one of the most common knee injuries. Partial meniscectomy and meniscal repair are the most common treatment options in the setting of an unstable meniscal tear. Standard MR diagnostic criteria of a meniscal tear may be normal findings postoperatively. The diagnosis of a recurrent or residual meniscal tear after prior meniscal surgery is primarily based on the visualization of surfacing high meniscal T2-weighted signal. After meniscectomy of greater than 25%, or meniscal repair, MR arthrography may be of benefit in the accurate evaluation of a possible residual or recurrent meniscal tear.

MAGNETIC RESONANCE IMAGING CLINICS OF NORTH AMERICA

SERIES OF RELATED INTEREST

Advances in Clinical Radiology
Neurologic Clinics
PET Clinics
Radiologic Clinics

VISIT THE CLINICS ONLINE!
Access your subscription at:
www.theclinics.com

PROGRAM OBJECTIVE
The goal of Magnetic Resonance Imaging Clinics of North America is to keep practicing physicians up to date with current clinical practice by providing timely articles reviewing the state of the art in patient care.

TARGET AUDIENCE
All practicing physicians and healthcare professionals who provide patient care utilizing findings from Magnetic Resonance Imaging.

LEARNING OBJECTIVES
Upon completion of this activity, participants will be able to:
1. Review the normal anatomy of the bone and soft tissue of the knee to further develop the necessary assessment skills needed to identify present and potential complications. Also, to assist in determining the appropriate use of MR imaging in diagnosing and treatment planning.
2. Discuss the variations of the bone and soft tissue of the knee requiring the use of MR imaging, with or without contrast and other diagnostic procedures, to assist in identifying present or potential complications, diagnosing and treatment planning, pre-or postoperatively.
3. Recognize the significance of MR imaging as a tool in guiding diagnosis, treatment planning, evaluation of treatment, grading of injuries, detecting and characterizing acute and chronic conditions, and promoting reduction of symptoms and restoration of function in all patient populations.

ACCREDITATION
The Elsevier Office of Continuing Medical Education (EOCME) is accredited by the Accreditation Council for Continuing Medical Education (ACCME) to provide continuing medical education for physicians.

The EOCME designates this journal-based CME activity enduring material for a maximum of 10 *AMA PRA Category 1 Credit*(s)™. Physicians should claim only the credit commensurate with the extent of their participation in the activity.

All other healthcare professionals requesting continuing education credit for this enduring material will be issued a certificate of participation.

DISCLOSURE OF CONFLICTS OF INTEREST
The EOCME assesses conflict of interest with its instructors, faculty, planners, and other individuals who are in a position to control the content of CME activities. All relevant conflicts of interest that are identified are thoroughly vetted by EOCME for fair balance, scientific objectivity, and patient care recommendations. EOCME is committed to providing its learners with CME activities that promote improvements or quality in healthcare and not a specific proprietary business or a commercial interest.

The planning committee, staff, authors and editors listed below have identified no financial relationships or relationships to products or devices they or their spouse/life partner have with commercial interest related to the content of this CME activity:
Erin Alaia, MD; Hamza Alizai, MD; Hailey Allen, MD; Connie Y. Chang, MD; Ceylan Colak, MD; Kirkland W. Davis, MD, FACR; Sonja Fierstra, MD; Donald Flemming, MD; Kara G. Gill, MD; Soterios Gyftopoulos, MD, MBA, MSc; Corey K. Ho, MD; MK Jesse, MD; William W. Kesler, MD; Iman Khodarahmi, MD, MSc, PhD; Pradeep Kuttysankaran; Alexander N. Merkle, MD; Megan K. Mills, MD; Lane Miner, DO; Mini N. Pathria, MD; Adam Rudd, MD; Lynne S. Steinbach, MD, FACR; Colin D. Strickland, MD; Naveen Subhas, MD, MPH; Doreen Thomas-Payne, MSN, BSN, RN, PMHNP-BC; Lukas M. Trunz, MD; John Vassallo; Joao R.T. Vicentini, MD; Armando F. Vidal, MD; Carissa M. White, MD; Lawrence M. White, MD, FRCPC; Fangbai Wu, MD

The planning committee, staff, authors and editors listed below have identified financial relationships or relationships to products or devices they or their spouse/life partner have with commercial interest related to the content of this CME activity:
William B. Morrison, MD, FACR: *Owner*: Trace Orthopedics; *Consultant*: Apriomed, Zimmer-Biomet Inc, Medical Metrics Inc; *Co-patent owner*: Apriomed

UNAPPROVED/OFF-LABEL USE DISCLOSURE
The EOCME requires CME faculty to disclose to the participants:
1. When products or procedures being discussed are off-label, unlabelled, experimental, and/or investigational (not US Food and Drug Administration [FDA] approved); and
2. Any limitations on the information presented, such as data that are preliminary or that represent ongoing research, interim analyses, and/or unsupported opinions. Faculty may discuss information about pharmaceutical agents that is outside of FDA-approved labelling. This information is intended solely for CME and is not intended to promote off-label use of these medications. If you have any questions, contact the medical affairs department of the manufacturer for the most recent prescribing information.

TO ENROLL

To enroll in the *Magnetic Resonance Imaging Clinics of North America* Continuing Medical Education program, call customer service at 1-800-654-2452 or sign up online at http://www.theclinics.com/home/cme. The CME program is available to subscribers for an additional annual fee of USD 281.00.

METHOD OF PARTICIPATION

In order to claim credit, participants must complete the following:

1. Complete enrolment as indicated above.
2. Read the activity.
3. Complete the CME Test and Evaluation. Participants must achieve a score of 70% on the test. All CME Tests and Evaluations must be completed online.

CME INQUIRIES/SPECIAL NEEDS

For all CME inquiries or special needs, please contact elsevierCME@elsevier.com.

Foreword
MR Imaging of the Knee

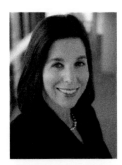

Lynne S. Steinbach, MD, FACR
Consulting Editor

Abbreviation	
MRI	magnetic resonance imaging

It is with great anticipation and excitement that I share this issue with you on the joint that made it all happen in the musculoskeletal MR imaging world. Of course, I am talking about the knee. Everyone thinks they can read a knee MRI and know all they need to about this important weight-bearing joint. As the years have gone by, there has been so much to learn about the knee. Research comes out every month that gives us new perspectives on knee injury patterns and MR imaging findings that open our eyes to better recognition, diagnosis, and treatment of associated disorders.

Who better to edit such an issue than a shining star who has risen in the world of musculoskeletal imaging and intervention: MK Jesse, MD. Dr Jesse hails from University of Colorado, where she is Chief of the Interventional Musculoskeletal Section. She has organized this issue into 10 timely topics written by esteemed leaders in the field.

Hot topics include findings in the posterolateral and posteromedial corners of the knee that can be easily overlooked, an update on cartilage injury and repair, plica and impingement syndromes, the newest information about preoperative and postoperative evaluation of the menisci and cruciate ligaments, synovitis and synovial pathologic conditions, bursae around the knee, pediatric normal variants, and neoplasms and masslike lesions.

A thank you to all the authors for putting together this incredible update of MR imaging of the knee during the trying times of the COVID Pandemic. This should serve as a new reference standard for knee imaging. Happy reading!

Lynne S. Steinbach, MD, FACR
Department of Radiology and Biomedical Imaging
University of California, San Francisco
505 Parnassus
San Francisco, CA 94143, USA

E-mail address:
lynne.steinbach@ucsf.edu

Magn Reson Imaging Clin N Am 30 (2022) xi
https://doi.org/10.1016/j.mric.2021.11.014
1064-9689/22/© 2021 Published by Elsevier Inc.

Preface
MR Imaging of the Knee

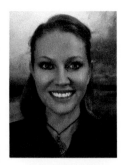

MK Jesse, MD
Editor

MR imaging is an invaluable tool in medical practice with an abundance of utilization in the field of orthopedics. Within the orthopedic subset, knee imaging is the most common and the accurate interpretation of knee MR is a necessary and critical tool for both the general and musculoskeletal radiologist. As our understanding of this complex joint increases, ultimately so does the expectation of the radiologist. We hope to narrow the inevitable time-related knowledge gaps through the comprehensive discussions presented in this issue.

This issue of Magnetic Resonance Imaging Clinics of North America focuses on the intricacies of diagnosis in MR imaging of the knee. Complex anatomy and pathologic conditions of meniscus, ligaments, and cartilage will be discussed along with up-to-date literature on the subtle secondary findings in internal derangement and other pathologic conditions. New advancements in the surgical treatment of meniscal tears, ligament pathology, and cartilage abnormalities create diagnostic challenges for radiologists. In this issue, our musculoskeletal radiology experts assist in the understanding of these new advancements and navigate the reader through the complex imaging features seen in each of these unique post-surgical cases.

In addition to the classic internal derangements of the knee, this issue will explore the new and exciting literature and imaging features of pathologic conditions of the knee bursa, plica, and fat pads as well as touch on the rare but important intra-articular and synovial pathologic conditions affecting the knee joint.

I am hopeful that this issue of Magnetic Resonance Imaging Clinics of North America will provide exciting new insights into MR imaging of the knee that may be used in everyday practice, teaching, and investigation.

MK Jesse, MD
Department of Radiology
University of Colorado Hospital
Anschutz Outpatient Pavilion
Department of Radiology
1635 Aurora Court
Aurora, CO 80045, USA

E-mail address:
mary.jesse@cuanschutz.edu

Magn Reson Imaging Clin N Am 30 (2022) xiii
https://doi.org/10.1016/j.mric.2021.11.013
1064-9689/22/© 2021 Published by Elsevier Inc.

MR Imaging of the Knee Posterolateral and Posteromedial Corner Injuries

Iman Khodarahmi, MD, MSc, PhD[a],*, Hamza Alizai, MD[b], Erin Alaia, MD[a], Soterios Gyftopoulos, MD, MBA, MSc[c]

KEYWORDS

• Knee MRI • Posterolateral • Posteromedial • Corner • Instability

KEY POINTS

- Injuries of the posteromedial and posterolateral corners of the knee are often present in patients with multiligamentous knee injuries but can be easily overlooked.
- Understanding of the anatomy, biomechanics, and typical imaging patterns of the posteromedial and posterolateral corners increases the chances of making an accurate diagnosis on MRI.
- Careful review and description of an injury in the posteromedial and posterolateral corners is needed to help the patient and provider make the most appropriate treatment decision.

INTRODUCTION

Injuries of the posteromedial (PMC) and posterolateral corners (PLC) of the knee are often present in patients with multiligamentous knee injuries but can be easily overlooked on imaging.[1,2] Untreated PMC injuries can lead to valgus and anteromedial rotatory instability,[3] whereas PLC injuries can lead to chronic posterolateral instability.[4] Secondary instabilities resulting from unrecognized PLC and PMC injuries can lead to significant morbidity including poor outcomes after anterior cruciate ligament (ACL) or posterior cruciate ligament (PCL) reconstruction.

After a knee injury, plain films and computed tomography can be useful for assessment of osseous abnormalities such as avulsion fractures. Stress radiographs may also be used for objective assessment of knee instability by measurement of the joint gap and comparison with the contralateral side.[5] Ultrasound has been found to be an expedient complementary modality for assessment of PLC[6] and can similarly be used for PMC but is operator dependent. Magnetic resonance imaging (MR imaging) provides an unparalleled multiplanar evaluation of knee soft tissues and is considered the reference standard. MR imaging advances continue to improve delineation and assessment of the intricate soft tissue-osseous relationships that make up the posteromedial and posterolateral corners and contribute to both static and dynamic stability of the knee joint.[7] The purpose of this narrative review is to describe the complex anatomy, biomechanics, injuries, and imaging appearance of the PMC and the PLC injuries.

POSTEROLATERAL CORNER
Normal Anatomy of the Posterolateral Corners

The PLC of the knee, once referred to as the "dark side" due to the limited understanding of the anatomic structures, may still pose a diagnostic challenge to radiologists and other clinicians. Based on our improved understanding of their biomechanics, PLC structures are grouped into primary (static) stabilizers and secondary (static

[a] Department of Radiology, NYU Langone Health, 660 1st Avenue, New York, NY 10016, USA; [b] Department of Radiology, Scottish Rite for Children, 2222 Welborn Street, Dallas, TX 75219, USA; [c] Departments of Radiology and Orthopedic Surgery, NYU Langone Health, 660 1st Avenue, New York, NY 10016, USA
* Corresponding author. Center for Biomedical Imaging, 660 1st Avenue, Room 223, New York, NY 10016.
E-mail address: Iman.Khodarahmi@nyulangone.org
Twitter: @IKhodarahmi (I.K.)

Magn Reson Imaging Clin N Am 30 (2022) 215–226
https://doi.org/10.1016/j.mric.2021.11.003
1064-9689/22/© 2021 Elsevier Inc. All rights reserved.

and dynamic) stabilizers. The fibular collateral ligament, popliteus tendon, and popliteofibular ligament are the 3 primary stabilizers of the PLC of the knee.[8]

Fibular collateral ligament

The fibular (lateral) collateral ligament (FCL) originates from a small bony depression slightly proximal and posterior to the lateral epicondyle and courses distally to insert on the fibular head distal to the tip of the fibular styloid (**Fig. 1**). The distal attachment may merge with the distal biceps femoris tendon to form a conjoined structure. On MR imaging, the FCL is best visualized on axial and coronal images as a low-signal-intensity band extending from the lateral aspect of the distal femur to the lateral aspect of the proximal fibula[9,10] (**Fig. 2A**).

Popliteus tendon

The popliteus tendon (PLT) originates from the anterior portion of the popliteus sulcus of the lateral femoral condyle, anterior to the FCL femoral attachment. It runs posteromedially deep to the FCL and exists the joint capsule through the popliteal hiatus (see **Fig. 1**). The popliteus myotendinous junction courses deep to the arcuate and fabellofibular ligaments (FFL) before the popliteus muscle inserts along the posteromedial aspect of the proximal tibia in an oblique fashion. On MR imaging, the PLT is seen as a low-signal-intensity structure on axial and sagittal images (**Fig. 2**). Anterior and posterior bundles of the PLT, which are taut in flexion and extension, respectively, may not be distinguished on imaging. Rarely, a

sesamoid bone, known as a cyamella, may be identified in the PLT.[10]

Popliteofibular ligament

The popliteofibular ligament (PFL) originates from PLT just proximal to the myotendinous junction, courses inferolaterally, and inserts onto the medial downslope of the fibular styloid (see **Fig. 1**). The anterior and posterior divisions of the PFL embrace the popliteus myotendinous junction.[9] On conventional MR imaging, the PFL is best seen as a low-T2-signal structure on coronal and sagittal MR images, deep to the inferior lateral genicular vessels. However, despite being present in 93% to 100% of cadaveric samples and having a cross-sectional area equal to that of the popliteus tendon, the PFL is difficult to identify with conventional MR imaging.[11,12] Improved visualization of the PFL has been reported with application of coronal oblique planes perpendicular to the PLT[13] and isotropic 3-dimensional pulse sequences[14] (see **Fig. 2**).

Secondary stabilizers

Secondary structures acting as static and dynamic stabilizers include the following:

- The midthird lateral capsular ligament is defined as thickening of the lateral capsule of the knee, which extends from the lateral epicondyle of the femur anterior to the origin of the lateral collateral ligament with capsular attachments to the lateral meniscus and inserts onto the tibia anterior to the popliteal hiatus.[15] This structure has been divided into meniscofemoral and meniscotibial ligaments and has

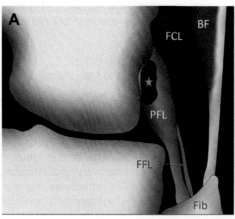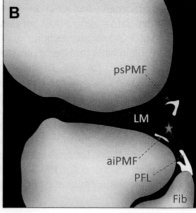

Fig. 1. Schematic illustrations of the posterolateral corner (PLC) of the knee. (A) Coronal view of the PLC shows the biceps femoris (BF) and fibular collateral ligament (FCL) along the lateral aspect of the knee and their conjoint insertion to the fibular (Fib) styloid. The popliteus tendon (star) with its inferomedial oblique course is seen in face. The popliteofibular ligament (PFL) extends from the popliteus tendon to the fibular styloid. The fabellofibular ligament (FFL) runs parallel to the FCL and inserts onto the fibular styloid process tip. (B) Sagittal view of the PLC demonstrates the posterosuperior popliteomeniscal fascicle (psPMF) and the anteroinferior popliteomeniscal fascicle (aiPMF) extending from the posterior horn of the lateral meniscus (LM) to the popliteus tendon (star) to form the roof and floor of the popliteus hiatus.

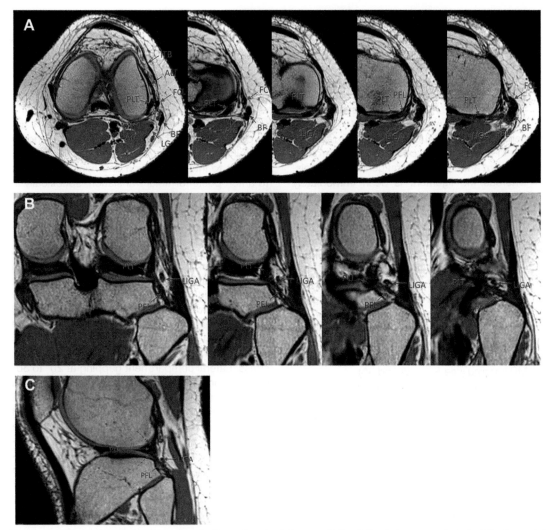

Fig. 2. Intermediate-weighted isotropic 3-dimensional MR images (0.5 × 0.5 × 0.5 mm voxel size) of the knee. (*A*) Axial knee images from proximal to distal (left to right) demonstrates various structures of the posterolateral corner, including the fibular collateral ligament (FCL), popliteus tendon (PLT), and popliteofibular ligament (PFL). Secondary stabilizers include the biceps femoris tendon (BF), the anterolateral ligament (ALT), lateral gastrocnemius tendon (LG), iliotibial band (ITB), and arcuate ligament (Arc). Note the anteromedial positioning of the PFL relative to the lateral inferior genicular artery (LIGA). (*B*) Coronal knee images from anterior to posterior (left to right) show the PFL extending from the PLT to the fibular styloid and its association with respect to the LIGA. (*C*) Sagittal lateral knee images show the PLT within the popliteus hiatus that is formed by the popliteomeniscal fascicles (*dashed arrows*) and the PFL located anterior to the LIGA.

been referred to as the anterolateral ligament of the knee in the recent literature[16,17] (see **Fig. 2A**).

- The popliteomeniscal fascicles connect the popliteus tendon to the posterior horn of the lateral meniscus and limit excessive motion of the lateral meniscus during knee extension. The posterosuperior and anteroinferior popliteomeniscal fascicles, seen on sagittal MR imaging, form the roof and floor of the popliteus hiatus, respectively[10] (see **Figs. 1** and **2C**).
- The lateral gastrocnemius tendon originates from the lateral femoral condyle about

14 mm posterior to the femoral FCL attachment. Injury to this tendon is less common than the other PLC structures[9] (see **Fig. 2A**).

- The FFL is the thickened distal aspect of the capsular arm of the short head of the biceps femoris that extends from an osseous fabella (or its cartilaginous analogue) to the fibular styloid. The fabella is a sesamoid bone within the proximal lateral gastrocnemius tendon found in 30% of individuals. The FFL runs parallel to the FCL and inserts onto the tip of the fibular styloid process, lateral to the attachment of the PFL and posterior to the attachment of the biceps femoris tendon[18] (see **Fig. 1** and **Fig. 3**). The inferior lateral genicular artery at the posterior joint capsule near the fibular styloid serves as a useful anatomic landmark, where it courses posterior to the PFL and anterior to the FFL.[19] Presence and visibility of the FFL is variable (visible in 33%–48% of patients).[20] On sagittal and coronal MR imaging, the FFL is best seen posterior to the arcuate ligament and inferior lateral genicular vessels, whereas the ligament is seen immediately anterior to the lateral head of the gastrocnemius tendon on axial images (see **Fig. 3**).

- The arcuate ligament is not considered a distinct anatomic structure by some investigators,[19] whereas others describe it as a Y-shaped thickening of the posterolateral joint capsule.[10,21] The arcuate ligament attaches to the fibular styloid with the FFL, lateral to the PFL.[18] Detection of the arcuate ligament is also inconsistent on imaging. It may seem as a thin low-signal-intensity band coalescing with the posterolateral capsule overlying the popliteus tendon on axial MR imaging (see **Figs. 2A and 3A**).
- The biceps femoris tendon consists of long and short heads. Distally each head is composed of at least 2 arms (direct and anterior). Except for the short head direct arm that passes medial to the FCL to insert onto the superolateral edge of the lateral tibial condyle, the remaining major arms insert onto the fibular head[10,22] (see **Fig. 2**). At MR imaging, the individual arms may not be easily distinguishable.
- The iliotibial band is a broad tendinous layer at the superficial aspect of the lateral knee, which inserts onto Gerdy tubercle at the anterolateral aspect of the tibia[9] (see **Fig. 2A**).

Biomechanics of the Posterolateral Corners

PLC structures serve as the primary restraints to knee varus stress and posterolateral rotation of the tibia with respect to the femur. They also act as secondary stabilizers to anterior and posterior tibial translation when cruciate ligaments are deficient.[23,24] To counteract a varus stress, the FCL acts as the primary stabilizer, whereas other PLC structures have a secondary role.[25] Regarding tibial external rotation, the FCL and the PLT act as primary stabilizers, and the PCL is a secondary restraint.[26] The PLC structures also provide minor restraint to internal rotation and minimal restraint to anteroposterior tibial translation, specifically in cruciate deficient knees.[9]

Clinical Presentation of Patients with Posterolateral Corner Injury

Patients often recall a specific trauma and complain of painful, difficulty walking on uneven surfaces, perceived sidewise instability near extension, or paresthesia/foot drop when the common peroneal nerve is damaged. Physical examination may reveal an abnormal varus stress test, defined as lateral compartment gapping with application of varus stress. Lateral compartment gapping at 20° to 30° knee flexion with restoration at knee full extension indicates an isolated injury to the FCL. Persistent gapping at full extension assumes a combined complex PLC and cruciate ligament injury. The dial test, reverse pivot shift test, and external rotation recurvatum test are other techniques to clinically evaluate the PLC.[9,21] Because of common associations, the physical examination should encompass evaluation of the cruciate ligaments, common peroneal nerve, and popliteal vessels.[27]

Posterolateral Corner Injuries and MR Imaging

Injuries to the PLC most commonly occur with varus forces particularly to a hyperextended knee. An expert consensus panel recommends MR imaging to always be performed in the assessment of suspected acute PLC injuries.[28] Injury to

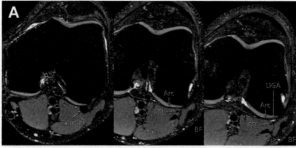
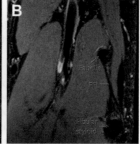

Fig. 3. Fat saturated T2-weighted isotropic 3-dimensional MR images (0.5 × 0.5 × 0.5 mm voxel size) of the knee. (*A*) Axial knee images from proximal to distal (left to right) demonstrate additional structure of the posterolateral corner, including the fabellofibular ligament (FFL) seen extending from the fabella to the fibular styloid, immediately anterior to the lateral gastrocnemius tendon (LG). Note the posterior location of the FFL relative to the lateral inferior genicular artery (LIGA). Arcuate ligament (Arc) and biceps femoris tendon (BF) are among the secondary stabilizers. (*B*) Coronal oblique view of the posterior knee shows the FFL throughout its course.

the FCL has been reported in 23% of patients who had posterolateral rotational instability at the time of surgery.[29] Such injuries can be easily identified on axial and coronal planes and range from periligamentous edema resulting from sprain to partial or complete tears to osseous avulsions in the acute setting (**Figs. 4–6**). A thickened ligament indicates chronic injury.

PLT injuries are classified as strains, partial tears, or complete tears with or without osseous avulsion fragments (see **Figs. 4, 6** and **7**). More commonly, the tears occur at the myotendinous junction where they are difficult to detect clinically due to accompanying injuries and arthroscopically owing to inherent difficulties in visualization of this area. Therefore, imaging plays a pivotal role in their detection. PFL injuries reflect as signal abnormality, tear, or avulsion from the fibular styloid process[10] (see **Figs. 4–7**). A sequential pattern of injury to the 3 major stabilizers of the PLC has been demonstrated, which include compromise of the FCL, followed by the PFL, and finally PLT, although there are exceptions (**Fig. 7**).

Assessing the FFL integrity is quite challenging. As other ligaments, FFL injuries may manifest as signal abnormality, tear, thickening, or avulsion. Such injuries often occur in conjunction with an avulsion injury of the short head direct arm of the biceps femoris tendon.[30] Pericapsular edema or capsular disruption at the posterolateral aspect of the joint suggests arcuate ligament injury (see **Figs. 4** and **5**). Biceps femoris tendon injuries are easily identified on MR imaging and are graded similar to tendons elsewhere (**Figs. 5** and **6**).

In regard to MR imaging diagnostic performance, a recent study on patients with acute ACL tear found complete tear or avulsion of the FCL was the most significant predictor of posterolateral instability, whereas assessment of the smaller PLC structures did not improve the diagnostic performance.[20]

Treatment of Posterolateral Corner Injuries

Current classification systems[31] of PLC injuries are too vague or complicated to be implementable in daily practice.[28] The Hughston grading system still forms the basis for treatment planning.[32] Grade I refers to sprain of PLC structures without varus or rotational instability. Grade II injury refers to partial PLC tear with slight or moderate varus or rotational laxity, and grade III injury reflects complete PLC tear with marked abnormal motion.

Grade I and II injuries are often treated nonoperatively, whereas grade III should be addressed surgically.[9,31] Surgery should be performed within 2 to 3 weeks following an acute injury. In chronic injuries, varus malalignment should be addressed with a high tibial osteotomy before or at the time of PLC reconstruction.

Concerning surgical techniques, primary stabilizer repair is a treatment option only in bone avulsions. Otherwise, the injured structure is reconstructed, while keeping uninjured structures untouched. Anatomic PLC reconstruction is reserved for patients in whom all primary PLC stabilizers are injured. One popular method of anatomic reconstruction is to use an Achilles allograft to reconstruct all 3 primary stabilizers, FCL, PLT, and PFL, through femoral, fibular, and tibial tunnels.[9] Hybrid procedures with reconstruction of primary and repair of secondary structures may also be performed.[28]

POSTEROMEDIAL CORNER
Normal Anatomy of the Posteromedial Corners

The PMC of the knee consists of ligaments, tendons, and capsular thickenings located between

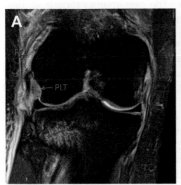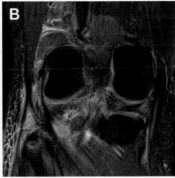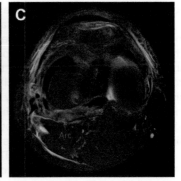

Fig. 4. Posterolateral corner injury in a 24-year-old patient with skiing accident. (*A*) Coronal fat-saturated T2-weighted MR knee image shows partial tears of the fibular collateral ligament (FCL) and popliteus tendon (PLT) proximally. (*B*) More posteriorly, coronal fat-saturated T2-weighted MR image demonstrates partial tear of the PLT myotendinous junction and popliteofibular ligament sprain (PFL). (*C*) Axial fat-saturated T2-weighted MR image shows complete arcuate ligament (Arc) tear. A torn anterior cruciate ligament is not included on these images.

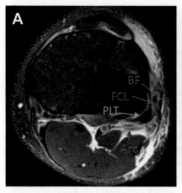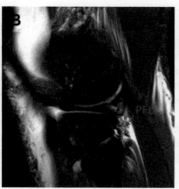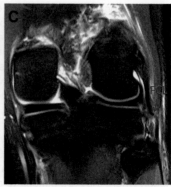

Fig. 5. Posterolateral corner injury in a 16-year-old patient with direct blow to the knee while playing soccer. (*A*) Axial fat-saturated T2-weighted MR knee image demonstrates fibular collateral ligament (FCL) complete tear, biceps femoris tendon (BF) split tear, and arcuate ligament (Arc) tear, whereas the popliteus tendon (PLT) remains intact. (*B*) Sagittal fat-saturated T2-weighted MR image shows popliteofibular ligament (PFL) partial tear. (*C*) Coronal fat-saturated T2-weighted MR image demonstrates FCL discontinuity. A torn anterior cruciate ligament is not shown on these images.

the superficial medial collateral ligament (sMCL) and the medial border of the PCL (**Fig. 8**). The PMC is discussed less frequently in radiology literature than the PLC; however, it is an important contributor to static and dynamic knee stability.[5] The structures included in the PMC include: the sMCL, deep medial collateral ligament (dMCL), posterior oblique ligament (POL), oblique popliteal ligament (OPL), the posteromedial joint capsule, semimembranosus, and the posterior horn of the medial meniscus.[1,5,33,34] Although not traditionally included in the PMC, an international expert consensus panel included the MCL as an important component of the PMC.[34]

Medial collateral ligament
The sMCL is the main medial support structure of the knee. Its single proximal attachment is located proximal and posterior to the medial epicondyle.[5] The sMCL has 2 distinct distal attachments: the proximal tibia soft tissue attachment and a distal tibia attachment. The proximal tibia attachment is 1 cm distal to the joint line on the anterior arm of the semimembranosus tendon, whereas the distal attachment is 6 cm distal to the joint line on the tibia. The dMCL is adherent to but separable from the sMCL. Its proximal attachment is 1 cm distal to that of sMCL and distally it attaches to the medial meniscus body with meniscofemoral ligament proximally and meniscotibial ligament distally. Further distally, it attaches to the tibia 3 to 4 cm distal to the joint line.[5] The sMCL and dMCL are best visualized on coronal and axial MR imaging (see **Fig. 8**).

Semimembranosus tendon
The semimembranosus tendon fans out distally with 5 distinct attachment arms: (1) the direct arm (primary attachment), (2) the anterior arm (tibial arm, pars reflexa), (3) the capsular arm, (4) the extension to the OPL, and (5) the inferior (popliteal) arm[1,33,35] (**Fig. 9**).

The main tendon bifurcates into the direct and anterior arms just below the joint line. The direct arm passes deep to the anterior arm and inserts on the posteromedial tibial condyle and attaches to the posterior aspect of the coronary ligament of the medial meniscus posterior horn. The anterior arm passes under the POL and inserts onto the medial tibia superior to the superficial MCL insertion. The OPL extension arises approximately 2 cm proximal to the main tendon bifurcation. The capsular arm joins the posteromedial capsule and the capsular portions of the POL and OPL. The inferior (popliteal) arm passes beneath the POL and attaches to the tibia just above the superficial MCL attachment.[33–35] The multiple attachments of the semimembranosus are vital to its role as a dynamic stabilizer. The semimembranosus is best seen on axial and coronal MR imaging.

Posterior oblique ligament
The POL has traditionally been described to originate from the adductor tubercle,[36] but recent studies have found its origin to be just distal and posterior to the tubercle.[37] Distally, the POL ligament has 3 arms: superficial, central, and capsular. The central arm, the thickest and most import of the 3, attaches to the posteromedial aspect of the medial meniscus and the adjacent posteromedial tibia. The capsular arm is continuous with the posterior joint capsule, whereas the superficial arm attaches to the semimembranosus tendon tibial insertion and blends with the posterior sMCL.[37] On MR imaging, the POL is best seen on axial images (see **Fig. 8**).

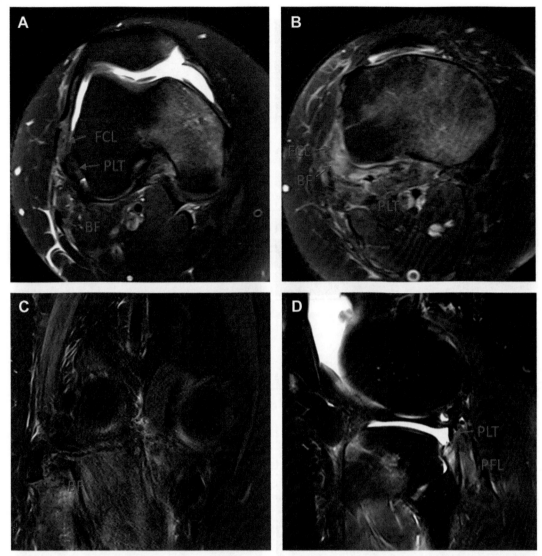

Fig. 6. Posterolateral corner injury in a 22-year-old patient with sport-related injury. (*A*) Axial fat-saturated T2-weighted MR knee image shows intact biceps femoris tendon (BF), fibular collateral ligament (FCL), partial tear, and popliteus tendon (PLT) strain. (*B*) Axial fat-saturated T2-weighted MR image at the level of the proximal tibia demonstrates complete BF and FCL tears and near-complete PLT myotendinous tear. (*C*) Coronal fat-saturated T2-weighted MR image depicts retraction of the torn BF. (*D*) Sagittal fat-saturated T2-weighted MR image shows popliteofibular ligament (PFL) sprain. A torn anterior cruciate ligament is not shown on these images.

Oblique popliteal ligament

The OPL is a component of both the PMC and PLC.[1] It arises from the POL capsular arm and semimembranosus lateral expansion and extends laterally and proximally toward the lateral femoral condyle.[1,33] At its lateral aspect, the OPL attaches to the meniscofemoral portion of the posterior joint capsule, an osseous or cartilaginous fabella, and to the plantaris muscle.[33,37] At MR imaging, OPL can be identified on all 3 planes (see **Fig. 8**).

Posteromedial joint capsule

The posteromedial joint capsule forms the dMCL with its meniscofemoral and meniscotibial components. Posteriorly, it is reinforced by the POL and semimembranosus expansions. It passes deep to the medial head of the gastrocnemius, extending laterally to join the posterior joint capsule. The posteromedial medial meniscus attaches to the capsule.[33,34] This structure is best seen on axial and sagittal MR imaging.

Posterior horn of the medial meniscus

The medial meniscus posterior horn is intimately associated with other PMC structures including the dMCL, POL, semimembranosus expansion, and the posteromedial capsule. Integrity of all these structures is important for a collective contribution

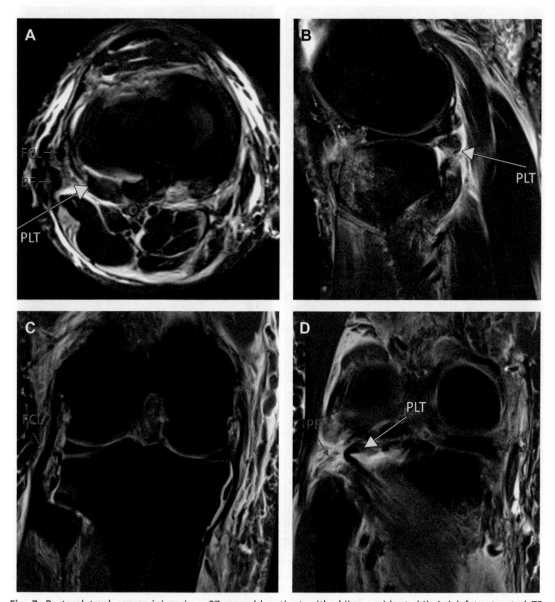

Fig. 7. Posterolateral corner injury in a 27-year-old patient with skiing accident. (*A*) Axial fat-saturated T2-weighted MR knee image shows intact biceps femoris tendon (BF) and fibular collateral ligament (FCL). The popliteus tendon (PLT) is completely torn and retracted. (*B*) Sagittal fat-saturated T2-weighted image demonstrates the retracted torn PLT. (*C, D*) Coronal fat-saturated T2-weighted MR images illustrate the intact FCL throughout its course, torn retracted PLT, and completely torn popliteofibular ligament (PFL). Torn anterior and posterior cruciate ligaments are not shown on these images.

to knee dynamic stability. Injury to the meniscotibial portion of the dMCL can cause meniscal instability, leading to increased stress on other PMC structures and further risk of injury[33] (see **Fig. 8**).

Biomechanics of the Posteromedial Corners

In terminal extension, the tibia rotates externally (screw-home movement), tightening the PMC. With flexion, the tibia rotates internally, whereas

the PMC progressively relaxes.[1] The sMCL, dMCL and POL are the main passive restraints of the PMC. The sMCL is the primary valgus restraint of the knee at all flexion angles as well as a stabilizer for external and internal rotation. The dMCL is secondary static restraint to valgus stress. The POL and the posteromedial capsule provide the primary valgus restraint at maximum extension. The POL is an important primary restraint to internal tibial rotation in an extended knee and

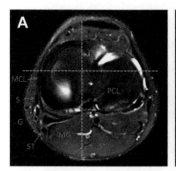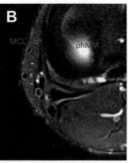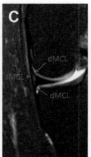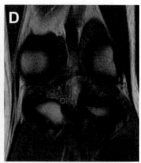

Fig. 8. (*A*) Axial fat-saturated T2-weighted MR knee image shows the posteromedial corner of the knee defined by the medial aspect of the posterior cruciate ligament (PCL) and anterior border of the medial collateral ligament (MCL) (*dashed lines*). Medial gastrocnemius (MG), semitendinosus (ST), gracilis (G), and sartorius (S) tendons are not among the posteromedial corner structures. (*B*) Magnified axial fat-saturated T2-weighted MR image of the posteromedial corner illustrates its contents, including the MCL, posterior oblique ligament (POL), semimembranosus tendon (SM), oblique popliteal ligament (OPL), and posterior horn of the medial meniscus (phMM). (*C*) Magnified coronal fat-saturated T2-weighted MR image of the medial knee shows the superficial (sMCL) and deep (dMCL) components of the MCL. (*D*) Coronal intermediate-weighted MR image through the posterior aspect of the femoral condyles demonstrate the oblique course of the OPL.

secondary stabilizer for valgus and external rotation.[33,34] The semimembranosus is a dynamic stabilizer: it acts as an active restraint to valgus when the knee is extended and as a restraint to external rotation when the knee is flexed.[1] It also places traction on the medial meniscus posterior horn, preventing meniscal injury from compression between the femur and tibia. The semimembranosus also places tension on and stabilizes the OPL and posteromedial capsule.[1] The OPL is the primary restrain to knee hyperextension.[38] A stable posterior horn of the medial meniscus with an intact meniscotibial ligament resists anterior tibial translation by engaging the posterior femoral condyle.[33] The PMC is also an important secondary stabilizer for anterior and posterior tibial translation. A compromised PMC can increase forces on ACL

and PCL, leading to graft failure after reconstructive surgery.[39]

Clinical Presentation of Patients with Posteromedial Corner Injury

These patients will present with pain, valgus instability, and anteromedial rotatory instability (AMRI).[34] The physical examination will generally reveal laxity (valgus gapping) with application of valgus stress, with the degree of laxity corresponding to the severity of PMC injury. In the presence of isolated sMCL tears, maximum laxity is at 20 to 30° of flexion. Valgus gapping observed at full extension may indicate injury of the dMCL, POL or both, and possible ACL injury. The anteromedial drawer test is used to assess anteromedial rotatory instability, and the dial test can be used to assess anteromedial tibial translation in the setting of PMC injury.[5]

Posteromedial Corner Injuries and MR Imaging

MR imaging is the modality of choice for assessment of PMC soft tissue injuries. Medial collateral ligament injuries are easily assessed on MR imaging and are graded as follows: grade I: microscopic tear manifesting with increased intrinsic signal on fluid-sensitive sequences and periligamentous edema; grade II: partial tear; and grade III: complete tear (**Figs. 10** and **11**). A study of patients with symptomatic AMRI found injury of the POL in 99% of the cases, injury to the semimembranosus in 70%, and peripheral meniscal detachment in 30%.[40] Semimembranosus tendon injuries may include partial tendon tears or avulsion fractures at its tibial attachment (direct arm insertion) (see **Fig. 11**). Complete tears of the

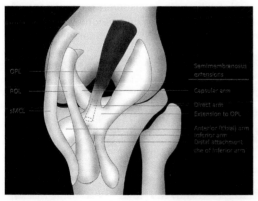

Fig. 9. Schematic illustrations of the posteromedial corner of the knee show 5 extensions of the semimembranosus tendon and their relation with adjacent structures: superficial medial collateral ligament (sMCL), posterior oblique ligament (POL), and oblique popliteal ligament (OPL).

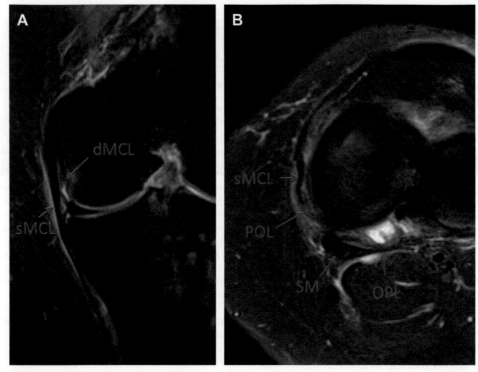

Fig. 10. Posteromedial corner injury in a 38-year-old patient with twisting knee injury. (*A*) Coronal fat-saturated T2-weighted MR knee image shows an intact superficial medial collateral ligament (sMCL) and deep medial collateral ligament (dMCL) sprain. (*B*) Axial fat-saturated T2-weighted MR image of the medial knee demonstrates posterior oblique ligament (OPL) partial tear, oblique popliteal ligament (OPL) sprain, and mild semimembranosus (SM) tendon strain. A torn anterior cruciate ligament is not shown on these images.

semimembranosus tendon are uncommon. POL injuries are graded using the same grading systems used for the MCL, and injuries may include low grade sprains, partial tears, and complete tears (see **Figs. 10** and **11**). Medial meniscocapsular injuries, particularly injuries of the meniscotibial ligament, can destabilize the meniscus increasing stress on other PMC structures. A "reverse Segond" fracture can be seen with meniscotibial ligament osseous avulsion, and this has a high association with PCL injury. OPL injuries may manifest with edema in the deep posteromedial aspect of the knee at the level of the joint line and irregularity of the OPL[41] (see **Figs. 10** and **11**).

Treatment of Posteromedial Corner Injuries

Combined rupture of the sMCL and POL with significant laxity in extended knee is predictive of residual laxity with conservative treatment. An international expert panel recommended treatment of isolated partial sMCL tears with a range

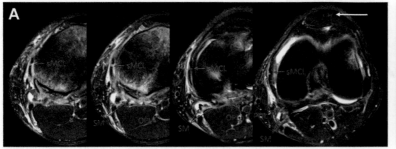
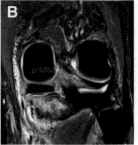

Fig. 11. Posteromedial corner injury in a 31-year-old patient with skiing accident. (*A*) Axial fat saturated T2-weighted MR images from proximal to distal (*right to left*) demonstrate superficial medial collateral ligament (sMCL) split tear, posterior oblique ligament (POL) partial tear, oblique popliteal ligament (POL) complete tear, and tear of the of the semimembranosus (SM) direct and anterior arms. The arrowhead in the far left image shows a cortical fragment related to osseous avulsion of the tibial arm of the SM. (*B*) Coronal fat-saturated T2-weighted MR image shows a radial tear at the posterior root of the medial meniscus (prMM).

of motion (ROM) brace.[34] This group, however, did not reach consensus regarding conservative (brace) versus surgical management of isolated grade III PMC injury (injury to sMCL, dMCL, and POL). They did suggest factors that may necessitate surgery with an isolated PMC injury include bony avulsions, intraarticular entrapment, or an MCL "stener-like" lesion.[34,42] The panel agreed that in the presence of a combined partial or complete PMC injury and ACL injury, the management should include an ROM brace followed by a delayed ACL reconstruction. Per this panel, if increased medial laxity is observed following the period of conservative treatment, then combined ACL and PMC reconstruction is indicated. Three ligament injuries (PMC, ACL, and PCL) should be managed with acute reconstruction. The overall goal of PMC reconstruction is to address valgus and rotational instability with anatomic reconstruction of the sMCL and POL recommended for chronic laxity. If valgus alignment on long-limb radiographs is observed in the context of chronic PMC laxity, alignment should be corrected before or simultaneously with PMC reconstruction.[34]

SUMMARY

The posteromedial and posterolateral corners of the knee are important areas to consider when assessing the patient with a possible knee injury. An understanding of the anatomy, associated biomechanics, and typical injury patterns in these regions allows the radiologist to provide the most comprehensive and useful MR interpretation ultimately improving patient care.

CLINICS CARE POINTS

- Injuries to the posterolateral corner of the knee commonly occur with varus forces particularly to a hyperextended knee.

- On MRI, injuries of the posterolateral corner of the knee often manifest as abnormalities of the fibular collateral ligament, popliteofibular ligament and popliteus tendon with the fibular collateral ligament being the most significant predictor.

- Patients with injuries of the posteromedial aspect of the knee present with pain, valgus instability and anteromedial rotatory instability.

- MRI is the modality of choice to identify posteromedial corner injuries. Failure to identify and address such injuries increases stress on the reconstructed cruciate ligaments, eventually leading to their failure.

DISCLOSURE

The authors have nothing to disclose.

REFERENCES

1. Lundquist RB, Matcuk GR Jr, Schein AJ, et al. Posteromedial corner of the knee: the neglected corner. Radiographics 2015;35(4):1123–37.
2. Temponi EF, de Carvalho Júnior LH, Saithna A, et al. Incidence and MRI characterization of the spectrum of posterolateral corner injuries occurring in association with ACL rupture. Skeletal Radiol 2017;46(8): 1063–70.
3. Tibor LM, Marchant MH Jr, Taylor DC, et al. Management of medial-sided knee injuries, part 2: posteromedial corner. Am J Sports Med 2011;39(6):1332–40.
4. Hughston JC, Jacobson KE. Chronic posterolateral rotatory instability of the knee. J Bone Joint Surg Am 1985;67(3):351–9.
5. Cinque ME, Chahla J, Kruckeberg BM, et al. Posteromedial corner knee injuries: diagnosis, management, and outcomes: a critical analysis review. JBJS Rev 2017;5(11):e4.
6. Sekiya JK, Swaringen JC, Wojtys EM, et al. Diagnostic ultrasound evaluation of posterolateral corner knee injuries. Arthroscopy 2010;26(4):494–9.
7. Khodarahmi I, Fritz J. The value of 3 tesla field strength for musculoskeletal MRI. Invest Radiol 2021;56(11):749–63.
8. LaPrade RF, Ly TV, Wentorf FA, et al. The posterolateral attachments of the knee: a qualitative and quantitative morphologic analysis of the fibular collateral ligament, popliteus tendon, popliteofibular ligament, and lateral gastrocnemius tendon. Am J Sports Med 2003;31(6):854–60.
9. Chahla J, Moatshe G, Dean CS, et al. Posterolateral corner of the knee: current concepts. Arch Bone Jt Surg 2016;4(2):97–103.
10. Rosas HG. Unraveling the posterolateral corner of the knee. Radiographics 2016;36(6):1776–91.
11. Watanabe Y, Moriya H, Takahashi K, et al. Functional anatomy of the posterolateral structures of the knee. Arthroscopy 1993;9(1):57–62.
12. Maynard MJ, Deng X, Wickiewicz TL, et al. The popliteofibular ligament. Rediscovery of a key element in posterolateral stability. Am J Sports Med 1996;24(3):311–6.
13. Yu JS, Salonen DC, Hodler J, et al. Posterolateral aspect of the knee: improved MR imaging with a coronal oblique technique. Radiology 1996;198(1): 199–204.
14. Rajeswaran G, Lee JC, Healy JC. MRI of the popliteofibular ligament: isotropic 3D WE-DESS versus coronal oblique fat-suppressed T2W MRI. Skeletal Radiol 2007;36(12):1141–6.
15. LaPrade RF, Gilbert TJ, Bollom TS, et al. The magnetic resonance imaging appearance of individual structures of the posterolateral knee. A prospective

study of normal knees and knees with surgically verified grade III injuries. Am J Sports Med 2000; 28(2):191–9.

16. Claes S, Vereecke E, Maes M, et al. Anatomy of the anterolateral ligament of the knee. J Anat 2013; 223(4):321–8.

17. Porrino J Jr, Maloney E, Richardson M, et al. The anterolateral ligament of the knee: MRI appearance, association with the Segond fracture, and historical perspective. AJR Am J Roentgenol 2015;204(2):367–73.

18. Pacholke DA, Helms CA. MRI of the posterolateral corner injury: a concise review. J Magn Reson Imaging 2007;26(2):250–5.

19. Moorman CT 3rd, LaPrade RF. Anatomy and biomechanics of the posterolateral corner of the knee. J Knee Surg 2005;18(2):137–45.

20. Filli L, Rosskopf AB, Sutter R, et al. MRI predictors of posterolateral corner instability: a decision tree analysis of patients with acute anterior cruciate ligament tear. Radiology 2018;289(1):170–80.

21. Covey DC. Injuries of the posterolateral corner of the knee. J Bone Joint Surg Am 2001;83(1):106–18.

22. Branch EA, Anz AW. Distal insertions of the biceps femoris: a quantitative analysis. Orthop J Sports Med 2015;3(9). 2325967115602255.

23. LaPrade RF, Tso A, Wentorf FA. Force measurements on the fibular collateral ligament, popliteofibular ligament, and popliteus tendon to applied loads. Am J Sports Med 2004;32(7):1695–701.

24. Grood ES, Stowers SF, Noyes FR. Limits of movement in the human knee. Effect of sectioning the posterior cruciate ligament and posterolateral structures. J Bone Joint Surg Am 1988;70(1): 88–97.

25. LaPrade RF, Wozniczka JK, Stellmaker MP, et al. Analysis of the static function of the popliteus tendon and evaluation of an anatomic reconstruction: the "fifth ligament" of the knee. Am J Sports Med 2010; 38(3):543–9.

26. Ranawat A, Baker CL 3rd, Henry S, et al. Posterolateral corner injury of the knee: evaluation and management. J Am Acad Orthop Surg 2008;16(9):506–18.

27. Essilfie AA, Alaia EF, Bloom DA, et al. Distal posterolateral corner injury in the setting of multiligament knee injury increases risk of common peroneal palsy. Knee Surg Sports Traumatol Arthrosc 2021.

28. Chahla J, Murray IR, Robinson J, et al. Posterolateral corner of the knee: an expert consensus statement on diagnosis, classification, treatment, and rehabilitation. Knee Surg Sports Traumatol Arthrosc 2019; 27(8):2520–9.

29. LaPrade RF, Terry GC. Injuries to the posterolateral aspect of the knee. Association of anatomic injury patterns with clinical instability. Am J Sports Med 1997;25(4):433–8.

30. Haims AH, Medvecky MJ, Pavlovich R Jr, et al. MR imaging of the anatomy of and injuries to the lateral and posterolateral aspects of the knee. AJR Am J Roentgenol 2003;180(3):647–53.

31. Shon OJ, Park JW, Kim BJ. Current concepts of posterolateral corner injuries of the knee. Knee Surg Relat Res 2017;29(4):256–68.

32. Hughston JC, Andrews JR, Cross MJ, et al. Classification of knee ligament instabilities. Part II. The lateral compartment. J Bone Joint Surg Am 1976;58(2):173–9.

33. Dold AP, Swensen S, Strauss E, et al. The Posteromedial corner of the knee: anatomy, pathology, and management strategies. J Am Acad Orthop Surg 2017;25(11):752–61.

34. Chahla J, Kunze KN, LaPrade RF, et al. The posteromedial corner of the knee: an international expert consensus statement on diagnosis, classification, treatment, and rehabilitation. Knee Surg Sports Traumatol Arthrosc 2020;29(9):2976–86.

35. Beltran J, Matityahu A, Hwang K, et al. The distal semimembranosus complex: normal MR anatomy, variants, biomechanics and pathology. Skeletal Radiol 2003;32(8):435–45.

36. Hughston JC, Eilers AF. The role of the posterior oblique ligament in repairs of acute medial (collateral) ligament tears of the knee. J Bone Joint Surg Am 1973;55(5):923–40.

37. LaPrade RF, Engebretsen AH, Ly TV, et al. The anatomy of the medial part of the knee. J Bone Joint Surg Am 2007;89(9):2000–10.

38. Morgan PM, LaPrade RF, Wentorf FA, et al. The role of the oblique popliteal ligament and other structures in preventing knee hyperextension. Am J Sports Med 2010;38(3):550–7.

39. LaPrade RF, Moulton SG, Nitri M, et al. Clinically relevant anatomy and what anatomic reconstruction means. Knee Surg Sports Traumatol Arthrosc 2015; 23(10):2950–9.

40. Sims WF, Jacobson KE. The posteromedial corner of the knee: medial-sided injury patterns revisited. Am J Sports Med 2004;32(2):337–45.

41. Geiger D, Chang E, Pathria M, et al. Posterolateral and posteromedial corner injuries of the knee. Radiol Clin North Am 2013;51(3):413–32.

42. Alaia EF, Rosenberg ZS, Alaia MJ. Stener-like lesions of the superficial medial collateral ligament of the knee: MRI features. AJR Am J Roentgenol 2019;213(6):W272–6.

MR Imaging of Knee Cartilage Injury and Repair Surgeries

Colin D. Strickland, MD[a],*, Corey K. Ho, MD[a], Alexander N. Merkle, MD[a],
Armando F. Vidal, MD[b]

KEYWORDS

• Cartilage • MRI • Microfracture • OATS • Allograft • ACI

KEY POINTS

- Fluid-sensitive fat-suppressed MR imaging may be used to assess morphologic cartilage defects and postoperative findings of cartilage repair.
- Debridement and microfracture techniques are performed with the goal of stimulating fibrocartilage formation at the site of cartilage damage.
- Numerous cartilage repair techniques including osteochondral allografting, autologous osteochondral transfer system (OATS), and autologous chondrocyte implantation (ACI) have been developed with the aim of reestablishing at least partial hyaline cartilage at the site of cartilage damage.
- Marrow edemalike signal may persist for months at sites of surgical cartilage repair. Fissuring, delamination, and lack of incorporation may signal failure of surgical cartilage repair.

INTRODUCTION

Articular cartilage injuries are a major source of morbidity and commonly coexist with other bone and soft tissue injuries at the knee. Hyaline cartilage has limited ability to heal following injury, which may lead to accelerated osteoarthritis, which is of particular concern in young athletes.[1,2] Both traumatic cartilage damage and accumulated chondral defects contribute to eventual loss of function and need for arthroplasty. Cartilage injuries are common, and a significant proportion encountered at arthroscopy may be amenable to surgical intervention.[3,4]

Cartilage injuries are commonly encountered by imagers, and several surgical treatment techniques have been developed. These techniques range from debridement and stimulated growth of fibrocartilage to allografting and autologous chondrocyte implantation (ACI). Newer techniques involve implantation of scaffolding material to provide structure and containment to chondrocyte substrates. The magnetic resonance (MR) imaging appearance of injured cartilage and regions of repair must be recognized by imagers to guide patient management and accurately predict clinical outcomes.

IMAGING OF ARTICULAR CARTILAGE

Articular cartilage is a mechanically critical component of the weight-bearing surface that distributes and dissipates force. Together with synovial fluid, the cartilage creates a near-frictionless surface for movement.[5] Cartilage consists of an extracellular matrix with associated fluid and a small percentage (by weight) of chondrocytes, which are responsible for maintaining homeostasis and generation of the macromolecular matrix.[6] A collagen matrix and proteoglycans, consisting of a protein with associated glucosaminoglycans (GAGs), provide mechanical structure. Typically

---

[a] Department of Radiology, University of Colorado School of Medicine, 12401 East 17th Avenue, Aurora, CO 80045, USA; [b] The Steadman Clinic and Steadman Philippon Research Institute, 181 West Meadow Drive, Suite 400, Vail, CO 81657, USA
* Corresponding author.
E-mail address: colin.strickland@cuanschutz.edu

Magn Reson Imaging Clin N Am 30 (2022) 227–239
https://doi.org/10.1016/j.mric.2021.11.004
1064-9689/22/© 2021 Elsevier Inc. All rights reserved.

trilaminar appearance of cartilage is described with a low-signal-intensity deep layer, a high-signal-intensity transitional layer, and a low-signal-intensity surface, although this appearance varies with the orientation of cartilage (and thus the constituent collagen network) to the main static magnetic field B_0.[7]

MR imaging provides excellent soft tissue contrast and resolution and is an invaluable tool for noninvasive evaluation of cartilage health and morphology. Clinical cartilage imaging is performed on high-field strength systems of at least 1.5 T (Tesla) and increasingly at 3 T. Use of a dedicated multichannel knee coil is also preferred for high-quality diagnostic imaging.

Typical conventional MR imaging sequences that assess morphologic defects may be used in the assessment of cartilage injuries and in the evaluation of postsurgical patients following cartilage repair. Two-dimensional (2D) fast spin echo (FSE) pulse sequences with intermediate proton density (PD) and/or T2 weighting in multiple planes are used due to high in-plane spatial resolution and additional utility in assessing other structures of the knee. Both 3-dimensional (3D) FSE pulse sequences and gradient echo sequences may be used to improve the spatial resolution and to evaluate the thickness and volume of cartilage at the expense of tissue contrast. Both 2D and 3D sequences can be used in the same protocol for complementary evaluation.

Beyond morphologic assessment, compositional MR imaging techniques are aimed at characterizing cartilage tissue and biochemical changes that occur before discrete defects (fissures and delamination, etc.) develop. As the collagen and GAG content of hyaline cartilage breaks down and becomes disorganized, permeability to water increases, creating physiologic differences that can be detected by MR imaging.[8] These differences can be detected by techniques such as quantitative T2 mapping, which has shown promise in the assessment of early cartilage degeneration and in monitoring following treatment. Studies have demonstrated the increased sensitivity in the detection of cartilage lesions when a T2 mapping sequence is added to a standard diagnostic protocol.[9] Correlation with progression of morphologic abnormalities has also been shown in patients with increased T2 values in articular cartilage over time.[10] T1ρ imaging, sodium imaging, and diffusion-weighted techniques are additional noninvasive techniques used in the evaluation of cartilage. Delayed gadolinium-enhanced MR imaging of cartilage (dGEMRIC) is a related technique that requires the intravenous administration of contrast followed by T1 mapping of cartilage.

These compositional techniques have yet to gain widespread clinical adoption due to challenging technical factors, specific software requirements, and lack of general expertise.[11]

IMAGING EVALUATION OF CARTILAGE INJURY

Cartilage damage may result from direct impact or shearing in the setting of an acute injury. Defects that arise in this manner are often sharply margin-ated (**Fig. 1**) and often demonstrate corresponding marrow edema or cortical fractures.[11] Chronic cartilage defects, on the other hand, tend to be more diffuse and with smooth, obtusely angulated margins (**Fig. 2**). Over time, chronic cartilage defects may be associated with changes to underlying bone with fracturing and remodeling of the subchondral bone plate.[12] Chronic defects are also typically multifocal and associated with secondary bony findings such as osteophyte formation and subchondral cystic change.

CARTILAGE INJURY CLASSIFICATION SYSTEMS

Several standardized grading systems exist for evaluation of morphologic cartilage defects. The Osteoarthritis Research Society International system is used extensively in research and describes the histopathologic features of cartilage defects of increasing severity.[12] The Outerbridge classification is widely accepted and used in the orthopedic community to facilitate communication between surgeons.[13] This classification is based on visual inspection and probing to characterize cartilage lesions. Grades include normal (grade 0), softening and swelling (grade I), partial-thickness fissures that do not reach bone and are less than 0.5 inches in diameter (grade II), partial-thickness fissures that reach bone and are greater than 0.5 inches in diameter (grade III), and erosion that exposes subchondral bone (grade IV). The International Cartilage Repair Society (ICRS) definitions are most widely used by imagers and closely parallel those in the Outerbridge classification (**Table 1**). ICRS grades include normal (grade 0), surface fibrillation or laceration (grade I), partial-thickness fissures that are less than 50% thickness (grade II), partial-thickness fissures that are greater than 50% thickness (grade III), and full-thickness defect with extension to subchondral bone (grade IV).[11]

CARTILAGE INJURY PATTERNS

Chondromalacia or softening may be difficult to detect on routine MR imaging evaluation. In the operating theater, the presence of cartilage

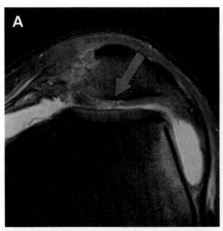
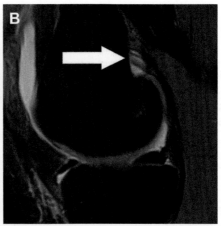

Fig. 1. Acute full-thickness cartilage defect at the patellar lateral facet (*red arrow*) on axial PD-weighted fat-saturated image (*A*) following transient patellar dislocation injury. The displaced cartilage fragment (*white arrow*) is visible on a sagittal PD-weighted fat-saturated image (*B*) deep to the medial gastrocnemius muscle origin.

softening is detected by direct probing during arthroscopic or direct surgical inspection. Increased signal on fluid-sensitive sequences may be noted on MR imaging, and elevated T2 values on T2 mapping correspond to these sites of early cartilage degeneration. Occasionally blistering of cartilage is also demonstrated, which may be visible as focal thickening of cartilage at the site of abnormal fluid retention. These sites may be asymptomatic at the time of clinical detection.

As cartilage damage progresses in severity, surface fibrillation and/or erosions may be detected on morphologic MR imaging sequences. The uneven superficial surface of cartilage is typically well demonstrated against the background of adjacent synovial fluid (**Fig. 3**). Cartilage thickness may be maintained or thinned in these regions. Fibrillation and erosion may be associated with formation of a cartilage flap in which a fissure propagates obliquely, deep to the articular surface, resulting in a potentially unstable defect. Cartilage may also separate entirely from the underlying bone plate with the potential to propagate and denude large regions of cartilage, particularly in the setting of additional shearing force. Dissection of fluid between cartilage and bone is typically well demonstrated by MR imaging depending on the orientation of the abnormality with respect to the plane of imaging.[14]

Cartilage thinning may be demonstrated by MR imaging, although variability in cartilage thickness exists among patients[15] and may even change dynamically in the minutes and hours following weight-bearing endurance exercise.[16] Focal areas of thinning, however, may be well demonstrated against the background of more normal adjacent articular cartilage.

Full-thickness cartilage defects are characterized by exposure of subchondral bone and are often accompanied by bony findings in the acute setting such as edema or fracture of the subchondral bone plate. Chronic full-thickness defects may demonstrate underlying bone sclerosis and central or intralesional osteophyte formation.[11]

CARTILAGE REPAIR TECHNIQUES

Numerous cartilage repair techniques exist, and the clinical practice of addressing cartilage defects has expanded to include a wide range of

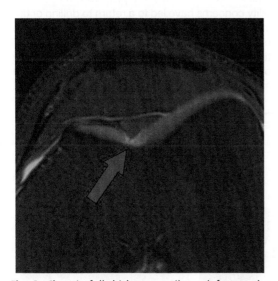

Fig. 2. Chronic full-thickness cartilage defect at the patellar medial facet (*red arrow*) on axial PD-weighted fat-saturated image. Note the rounded margins.

Table 1
Cartilage lesion grading systems

Grade	
Outerbridge Classification System	
0	Normal
I	Softening and swelling
II	Partial-thickness fissures that do not reach bone and are <0.5 in in diameter
III	Partial-thickness fissures that reach bone and are >0.5 in in diameter
IV	Erosion that exposes subchondral bone
ICRS Classification System	
0	Normal
1	Surface fibrillation or laceration
2	Partial-thickness fissures that are <50% thickness
3	Partial-thickness fissures that are >50% thickness
4	Full-thickness defect with extension to subchondral bone

new and innovative techniques. Early techniques were aimed at stimulating the growth of fibrocartilage at sites of damage, whereas more recent surgical approaches seek to replace regions of damaged cartilage by way of grafting or by fostering growth of a higher content of hyaline cartilage at the site of repair.

DEBRIDEMENT, ABRASION, AND DRILLING

Debridement of mechanically unstable cartilage defects may be used in isolation or as part of a more complex surgical intervention to address internal derangement. Cartilage flaps and foci of delamination are debrided with the goal of preventing propagation of further cartilage damage and the generation of intra-articular chondral or osteochondral bodies. In preparation for subsequent drilling or microfracture, the periphery of the defect is debrided to create vertical walls of surrounding cartilage to contain blood clot formation. The calcified layer of cartilage must be removed as well to ensure adherence of the clot to the bone surface.[17]

Abrasion and drilling of subchondral bone is then performed to stimulate bleeding and concomitant release mesenchymal stem cells and growth factors into a cartilage defect. A motorized drill to perforate the subchondral bone was used extensively in past decades, although concerns about thermal necrosis caused a decline in clinical use.[18]

MICROFRACTURE

Formation of a blood clot in the chondral defect and eventual maturation to fibrocartilage is the goal of the microfracture procedure.[19] Rather than use of a mechanical drill, a conical awl is used to perforate the bone resulting in small holes 2 to 4 mm in depth that are 3 to 4 mm apart (**Fig. 4**).[20] Despite the formation of fibrocartilage rather than hyaline cartilage, many patients report at least short-term clinical improvement.[21] Outcome data support the use of microfracture techniques in young patients with small defects (<2 cm^2).[21,22] Over time, however, fibrocartilage does not display the same durability as hyaline cartilage and progressive loss of joint function is typically seen.[23,24] In some practices, these durability concerns have led to a return to drilling or using microfracture only as a complement to a more extensive cartilage repair technique. Augmentation of microfracture with implantation of a variety of scaffolds (ranging from hyaluronic acid and atelocollagen-based scaffolds to denatured

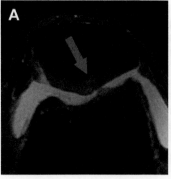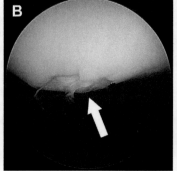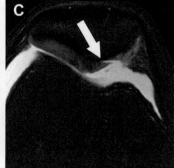

Fig. 3. Deep partial-thickness cartilage defect at the patellar median ridge (*red arrow*) on axial PD-weighted fat-saturated image (*A*) and at arthroscopy (*white arrow*) (*B*). Full-thickness cartilage fissure with associated flap formation (*white arrow*) on axial PD-weighted fat-saturated image (*C*).

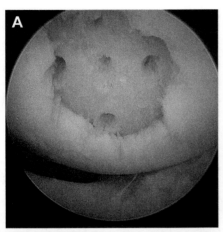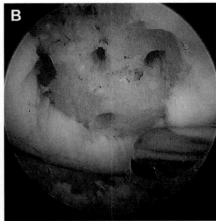

Fig. 4. Microfracture procedure with arthroscopic debridement of articular cartilage to a vertical edge with removal of the calcified cartilage layer and perforation of bone (*A*). Early bleeding and subsequent clot formation (*B*) will be followed by fibrocartilage formation.

fibrinogen) has shown promise in animal models and in early clinical case series.[25]

OSTEOCHONDRAL ALLOGRAFT

Large cartilage defects that may not be suitable for treatment with microfracture or drilling may be addressed by osteochondral allografting. This surgical approach is often used to address large cartilage lesions that involve the margin of an articular surface or an area of multiple adjacent defects. Osteochondral allografting is also used as a salvage procedure following failure of other previously attempted techniques.

Fresh cadaveric graft material is preferred with the goal of implantation as soon as possible following all appropriate screening and testing of the donor tissue. At the donor site, bone is debrided to a depth of 6 to 8 mm and a dowel- or shell-shaped implant (**Fig. 5**) is placed to best estimate the site and contour of the area to be treated.[26,27] Press-fit or bioabsorbable pin fixation is used to secure the graft. Surgical techniques and specialized instruments have been developed to minimize mechanical trauma to the graft during surgical implantation to maintain maximal chondrocyte viability.[28]

OSTEOCHONDRAL AUTOGRAFT TRANSFER SYSTEM OR MOSAICPLASTY

Transplantation of osteochondral tissue (in the form of small conical plugs of cartilage and underlying bone) from relatively non-weight-bearing regions of the knee is another surgical approach (**Fig. 6**). Mosaicplasty or osteochondral autograft transfer system (OATS) offers the advantage of replacing hyaline cartilage and underlying bone

at the site of injury. The procedure avoids the general risks of implanting allograft material and is associated with less immune response complications leading to graft failure, which may occur despite the absence of requirement for donor blood/human leukocyte antigen matching or immunosuppression in osteochondral allograft transplantation.[29] The procedure does, however, require the harvesting of autograft material from relatively non-weight-bearing regions of cartilage (such as the periphery of the trochlear articular surface) and carries with it the potential for donor site complications. The amount of autograft that may be harvested is also limited, and thus the technique is typically restricted to smaller defects (<4 cm^2).[30,31]

AUTOLOGOUS CHONDROCYTE IMPLANTATION

Initial techniques for cell-based cartilage repair were introduced in the 1990s and consisted of harvesting of chondrocytes from non-weight-bearing cartilage.[32] Harvested cells were then grown in culture for 3 to 5 weeks. The target cartilage defect was debrided and covered with a periosteal flap with the chondrocyte culture then injected underneath followed by a period of non-weight-bearing (**Fig. 7**). During this period, a hyalinelike articular cartilage formed as the injected chondrocytes formed a surrounding extracellular matrix.[32,33] The procedure has been shown to give significant functional improvement at 3 years and is associated with minimal donor site complications.[34,35] ACI may be used for large cartilage defects measuring 2 to 12 cm^2.[24,36,37] Complications include graft hypertrophy, arthrofibrosis, and failure of the periosteal flap.[36–39]

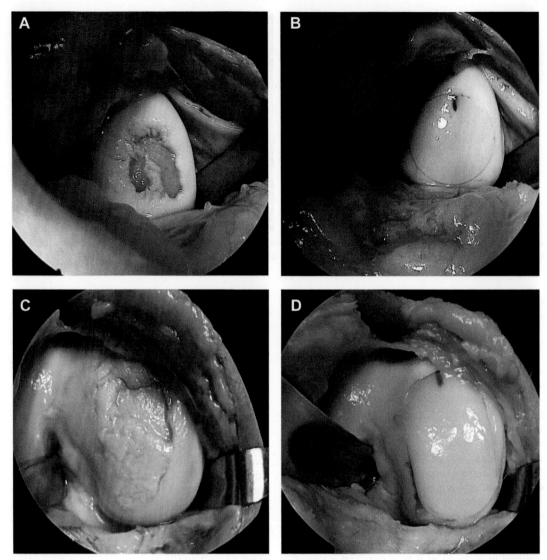

Fig. 5. Allograft procedure with intraoperative visualization of a full-thickness chondral defect (*A*) and subsequent grafting with a dowel-shaped implant (*B*). Large full-thickness defects (*C*) may also be addressed using a larger oval-shaped implant to match the curvature of the articular surface (*D*).

Modifications and variations of the ACI cell-based cartilage repair technique led to the evolution of the procedure, and ACI was subsequently supplanted by current matrix-assisted chondrocyte implantation (MACI) techniques. Early versions of MACI involved implantation of a porcine collagen membrane seeded with autologous chondrocytes in place of the periosteal flap and injected culture.[40] Initial clinical outcomes have been positive on long-term follow-up.[41]

Emerging techniques in cartilage repair include the implantation of biodegradable scaffold materials that may be shaped to precisely address cartilage defects and are implanted at the sites of microfracture.[25,42,43] These scaffolds may contain cartilage matrix components and growth factors aimed at stimulation of hyalinelike cartilage growth without the need for harvesting and culturing autologous chondrocytes.

MAGNETIC RESONANCE IMAGING OF REPAIRED CARTILAGE

MR imaging is the imaging modality of choice in the assessment of cartilage following surgical repair. Reparative cartilage is well depicted, as are the surrounding native articular surfaces and underlying bone. The standard clinical imaging

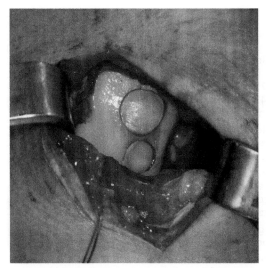

Fig. 6. OATS procedure with intraoperative visualization of 2 small plugs transferred from relatively non-weight-bearing bone in the same knee to treat small femoral condylar articular cartilage defects.

fissuring at the margins of repaired cartilage should also be assessed. Status of the underlying bone is also evaluated because edema and cyst formation may indicate evidence of treatment failure. To standardize and facilitate reproducible reporting, Magnetic Resonance Observation of Cartilage Repair Tissue (MOCART) scoring was introduced and based on a series of 9 variables.[46,47] Recently a modified and refined MOCART 2.0 scoring system and atlas were introduced to guide clinical reporting and standardized imaging research on cartilage repair.[48,49] This updated scoring system assesses 7 imaging features with variable point scales providing a single comprehensive score reflecting the health and integrity of repaired cartilage (**Table 2**). Additional semiquantitative reporting systems exist, including Cartilage Repair OA Knee Score (CROAKS), which incorporates some features of the MOCART system as well as cataloging other features in the treated knee, including the status of menisci, synovitis, and effusion.[50]

protocols may be used with intermediate-weighted FSE sequences constituting the primary imaging technique.[29] Compositional techniques including dGEMRIC, T1ρ, diffusion-weighted imaging, sodium MR imaging, and T2 mapping are also used at some centers. A 3-T system is preferred for a high signal-to-noise ratio and spatial resolution.[44] Heterogeneous signal characteristics may be observed in reparative cartilage due to the disorganization of collagen fibers when compared with native hyaline cartilage.[45]

Morphologic features of repaired cartilage are well demonstrated with MR imaging. The degree of filling of a chondral defect should be reported along with any possible graft hypertrophy. Any

IMAGING APPEARANCE FOLLOWING MICROFRACTURE

Complete cellular differentiation and fibrocartilage filling of defects treated with microfracture may take months to years.[51] Fibrocartilage forming at the site of microfracture initially may appear thin and demonstrate hyperintense signal on fluid-sensitive sequences, reflecting the disorganized matrix and high water permeability.[24,51] As fibrocartilage tissue matures it may take on a hypointense appearance on fluid-sensitive sequences (**Fig. 8**) and should eventually achieve a smooth, well-defined surface.[24,44] Defects that remain poorly filled and/or integrated or demonstrate

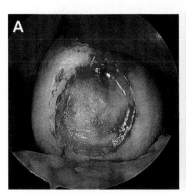
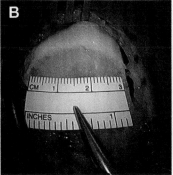
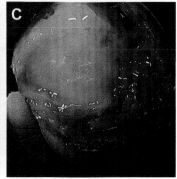

Fig. 7. ACI procedure with intraoperative visualization of a large lateral femoral condylar cartilage defect (*A*). The defect is debrided and measured (*B*) followed by coverage with periosteal flap under which a chondrocyte culture (grown from chondrocytes obtained from cartilage in same knee approximately 1 month before) is injected (*C*).

Table 2
MOCART 2.0 knee score: cartilage repair tissue assessment summarized features

Volume fill of cartilage defect	Complete or minor hypertrophy
	Major hypertrophy
	50%–75% filling of total defect
	25%–49% filling of total defect
	<25% filling of total defect or complete delamination
Integration into adjacent cartilage	Complete integration
	Splitlike defect at interface ≤2 mm
	Defect at interface >2 mm, but ≤50% of repair length
	Defect at interface >50% of repair length
Surface of the repair tissue	Surface intact
	Surface irregular ≤50% of repair tissue diameter
	Surface irregular >50% of repair tissue diameter
Structure of the repair tissue	Homogeneous
	Inhomogeneous
Signal intensity of the repair tissue	Normal
	Minor abnormal (hyperintense or hypointense)
	Severely abnormal (hyperintense or hypointense)
Bony defect or bony overgrowth	No defect or overgrowth
	Bony defect: depth < thickness of cartilage or overgrowth <50% of adjacent cartilage
	Bony defect: depth ≥ thickness of cartilage or overgrowth ≥50% of adjacent cartilage
Subchondral changes	No major subchondral changes
	Minor edemalike marrow signal <50% of repair tissue diameter
	Severe edemalike marrow signal ≥50% of repair tissue diameter
	Subchondral cyst ≥5 mm in longest diameter or osteonecrosislike signal

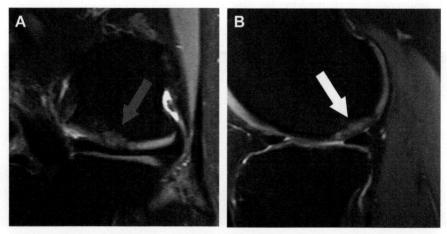

Fig. 8. Coronal (*A*) and sagittal (*B*) PD-weighted fat-saturated images demonstrating a mature lateral femoral condylar defect (*red arrow*) treated with microfracture. Note the heterogeneous appearance of fibrocartilage filling the defect compared with adjacent hyaline cartilage. Despite irregularity of the underlying subchondral bone plate, the articular surface is smooth and intact (*white arrow*).

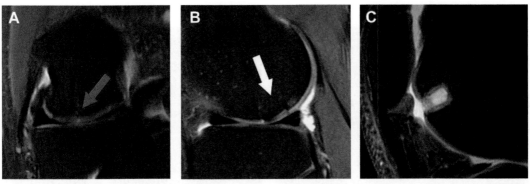

Fig. 9. Coronal (*A*) and sagittal (*B*) PD-weighted fat-saturated images demonstrating a lateral femoral condylar defect treated with OATS. Minimal marrow edemalike signal is demonstrated (*red arrow*); however, there is no cartilage fissuring or delamination. Note that the osteochondral graft is positioned such that the cartilage surface is smooth, which may leave a perceptible but clinically unimportant step-off along the contours of the subchondral bone at the fragment-native bone interface (*white arrow*). A defect from the trochlear harvest site remains visible on sagittal PD-weighted fat-saturated imaging (*C*).

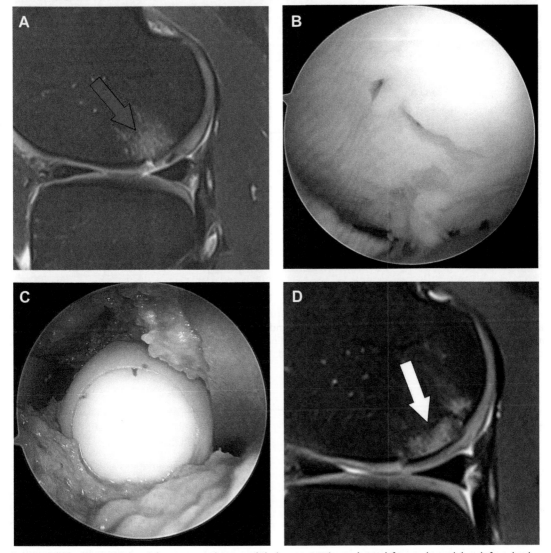

Fig. 10. Sagittal PD-weighted fat-saturated image (*A*) demonstrating a lateral femoral condylar defect (*red arrow*). Arthroscopic visualization demonstrates full-thickness cartilage damage (*B*) that was subsequently treated with an osteochondral allograft (*C*). Sagittal PD-weighted fat-saturated image (*D*) demonstrating the allograft in appropriate position with mild marrow edemalike signal (*white arrow*) within the graft, which may persist for up to 12 months.

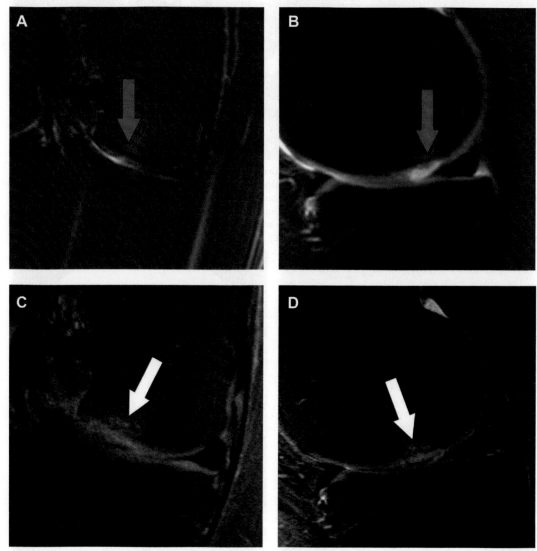

Fig. 11. Coronal (*A*) and sagittal (*B*) PD-weighted fat-saturated images demonstrating a region of full-thickness cartilage damage (*red arrows*) at the medial femoral condyle. Coronal (*C*) and sagittal (*D*) PD-weighted fat-saturated images obtained following ACI demonstrate hyaline cartilagelike tissue filling the defect (*white arrows*). Following ACI, the defect may appear slightly overfilled.

underlying marrow edemalike signal are associated with poor clinical outcomes.[21,24]

IMAGING APPEARANCE FOLLOWING ALLOGRAFTING

The superficial interface between the allograft and native cartilage should be smooth and follow the expected contour of the articular surface (**Fig. 9**). Bone surfaces should also be well approximated. Marrow edema in surrounding bone is common in the first few months following surgery but should resolve by 12 months.[44,51]

IMAGING APPEARANCE FOLLOWING OSTEOCHONDRAL AUTOGRAFT TRANSFER SYSTEM OR MOSAICPLASTY

Early postoperative imaging should demonstrate complete filling of the treated defect with matching of the articular surface contour between grafted and native cartilage.[52] Marrow edema within grafted and surrounding bone is commonly seen for up to 1 year, although over time the osteochondral bone plugs become indiscernible from the surrounding tissue. Cystic changes or persistent marrow edemalike signal may indicate graft failure.[24] It is important to note that the subchondral bone plate may be incongruous at the interface between grafted and adjacent bone, reflecting differences in cartilage thickness between the repaired site and donor site and the need to make the articular surface flush at the time of surgical implantation (**Fig. 10**).[51] Donor sites are often left unfilled at surgery and typically fill in with bone, although a residual defect typically remains visible at MR imaging.

MAGNETIC RESONANCE IMAGING OF AUTOLOGOUS CHONDROCYTE IMPLANTATION AND MATRIX-ASSISTED CHONDROCYTE IMPLANTATION

Reparative cartilage forming following an ACI or MACI procedure is initially hyperintense on fluid-sensitive sequences and evolves to resemble native cartilage in signal intensity over the course of a year following surgery (**Fig. 11**).[53] Surrounding marrow edemalike signal may be seen, which also resolves over time with persistence beyond 1 year, a sign of possible treatment failure.[24] Depending on the type of procedure performed, the treated area may initially be slightly overfilled (ACI) or appear underfilled (MACI). The interface between the repair and native cartilage should become less conspicuous over time, whereas linear increased fluid signal intensity undermining the base of reparative cartilage and bone suggests incomplete incorporation. Missing portions of repair tissue may also be seen in the setting of partial or complete repair failure.[24]

SUMMARY

Cartilage injuries are common and may predispose to early accelerated osteoarthritis. MR imaging is critical in the detection and characterization of injuries and guides treatments aimed at reducing symptoms, restoring function, and delaying arthroplasty. As the number of cartilage repair strategies has expanded, it is important that imagers understand the expected appearance of treated cartilage lesions and are positioned to detect complications that may require additional surgical intervention. Morphologic imaging features of cartilage damage and repair surgeries are well described, and several scoring systems have been developed to standardize evaluation in clinical trials and in clinical practice. Compositional MR imaging techniques provide additional microstructural assessment and will likely gain more widespread use as clinical experience is developed and they become more automated and time efficient.

CLINICS CARE POINTS

- Fluid-sensitive fat-suppressed MR imaging may be used to assess morphologic cartilage defects and postoperative findings of cartilage repair.
- Debridement and microfracture techniques are performed with the goal of stimulating fibrocartilage formation at the site of cartilage damage.
- Numerous cartilage repair techniques including osteochondral allografting, autologous osteochondral transfer system (OATS), and autologous chondrocyte implantation (ACI) have been developed with the aim of reestablishing at least partial hyaline cartilage at the site of cartilage damage.
- Marrow edemalike signal may persist for months at sites of surgical cartilage repair. Fissuring, delamination, and lack of incorporation may signal failure of surgical cartilage repair.

DISCLOSURE

A.F. Vidal discloses that he is on the Board of the American Academy of Orthopedic Surgeons. The authors have no financial disclosures.

REFERENCES

1. Bay-Jensen AC, Hoegh-Madsen S, Dam E, et al. Which elements are involved in reversible and irreversible cartilage degradation in osteoarthritis? Rheumatol Int 2010;30(4):435–42.
2. Messner K, Maletius W. The long-term prognosis for severe damage to weight-bearing cartilage in the knee: a 14-year clinical and radiographic follow-up in 28 young athletes. Acta Orthop Scand 1996; 67(2):165–8.
3. Aroen A, Loken S, Heir S, et al. Articular cartilage lesions in 993 consecutive knee arthroscopies. Am J Sports Med 2004;32(1):211–5.
4. Curl WW, Krome J, Gordon ES, et al. Cartilage injuries: a review of 31,516 knee arthroscopies. Arthroscopy 1997;13(4):456–60.
5. Huber M, Trattnig S, Lintner F. Anatomy, biochemistry, and physiology of articular cartilage. Invest Radiol 2000;35(10):573–80.
6. Burstein D, Gray M, Mosher T, et al. Measures of molecular composition and structure in osteoarthritis. Radiol Clin North Am 2009;47(4):675–86.
7. Goodwin DW, Zhu H, Dunn JF. In vitro MR imaging of hyaline cartilage: correlation with scanning electron

microscopy. AJR Am J Roentgenol 2000;174(2): 405–9.

8. Binks DA, Hodgson RJ, Ries ME, et al. Quantitative parametric MRI of articular cartilage: a review of progress and open challenges. Br J Radiol 2013; 86(1023):20120163.

9. Kijowski R, Blankenbaker DG, Munoz Del Rio A, et al. Evaluation of the articular cartilage of the knee joint: value of adding a T2 mapping sequence to a routine MR imaging protocol. Radiology 2013; 267(2):503–13.

10. Pan J, Pialat JB, Joseph T, et al. Knee cartilage T2 characteristics and evolution in relation to morphologic abnormalities detected at 3-T MR imaging: a longitudinal study of the normal control cohort from the Osteoarthritis Initiative. Radiology 2011;261(2):507–15.

11. Komarraju A, Goldberg-Stein S, Pederson R, et al. Spectrum of common and uncommon causes of knee joint hyaline cartilage degeneration and their key imaging features. Eur J Radiol 2020;129: 109097.

12. Pritzker KP, Gay S, Jimenez SA, et al. Osteoarthritis cartilage histopathology: grading and staging. Osteoarthritis Cartilage 2006;14(1):13–29.

13. Slattery C, Kweon CY. Classifications in brief: outerbridge classification of chondral lesions. Clin Orthop Relat Res 2018;476(10):2101–4.

14. Kendell SD, Helms CA, Rampton JW, et al. MRI appearance of chondral delamination injuries of the knee. AJR Am J Roentgenol 2005;184(5):1486–9.

15. Eckstein F, Winzheimer M, Hohe J, et al. Interindividual variability and correlation among morphological parameters of knee joint cartilage plates: analysis with three-dimensional MR imaging. Osteoarthritis Cartilage 2001;9(2):101–11.

16. Kessler MA, Glaser C, Tittel S, et al. Recovery of the menisci and articular cartilage of runners after cessation of exercise: additional aspects of in vivo investigation based on 3-dimensional magnetic resonance imaging. Am J Sports Med 2008;36(5): 966–70.

17. York PJ, Wydra FB, Belton ME, et al. Joint preservation techniques in orthopaedic surgery. Sports Health 2017;9(6):545–54.

18. Kraeutler MJ, Aliberti GM, Scillia AJ, et al. Microfracture versus drilling of articular cartilage defects: a systematic review of the basic science evidence. Orthop J Sports Med 2020;8(8). 2325967120945313.

19. Gracitelli GC, Moraes VY, Franciozi CE, et al. Surgical interventions (microfracture, drilling, mosaicplasty, and allograft transplantation) for treating isolated cartilage defects of the knee in adults. Cochrane Database Syst Rev 2016;9:CD010675.

20. Mithoefer K, Williams RJ 3rd, Warren RF, et al. The microfracture technique for the treatment of articular cartilage lesions in the knee. A prospective cohort study. J Bone Joint Surg Am 2005;87(9):1911–20.

21. Mithoefer K, McAdams T, Williams RJ, et al. Clinical efficacy of the microfracture technique for articular cartilage repair in the knee: an evidence-based systematic analysis. Am J Sports Med 2009;37(10): 2053–63.

22. Bae DK, Yoon KH, Song SJ. Cartilage healing after microfracture in osteoarthritic knees. Arthroscopy 2006;22(4):367–74.

23. Smith GD, Knutsen G, Richardson JB. A clinical review of cartilage repair techniques. J Bone Joint Surg Br 2005;87(4):445–9.

24. Alparslan L, Winalski CS, Boutin RD, et al. Postoperative magnetic resonance imaging of articular cartilage repair. Semin Musculoskelet Radiol 2001;5(4):345–63.

25. Shah SS, Lee S, Mithoefer K. Next-generation marrow stimulation technology for cartilage repair: basic science to clinical application. JBJS Rev 2021;9(1):e20 00090.

26. Sherman SL, Garrity J, Bauer K, et al. Fresh osteochondral allograft transplantation for the knee: current concepts. J Am Acad Orthop Surg 2014; 22(2):121–33.

27. Murphy RT, Pennock AT, Bugbee WD. Osteochondral allograft transplantation of the knee in the pediatric and adolescent population. Am J Sports Med 2014;42(3):635–40.

28. Bugbee WD, Pallante-Kichura AL, Gortz S, et al. Osteochondral allograft transplantation in cartilage repair: Graft storage paradigm, translational models, and clinical applications. J Orthop Res 2016;34(1):31–8.

29. Liu YW, Tran MD, Skalski MR, et al. MR imaging of cartilage repair surgery of the knee. Clin Imaging 2019;58:129–39.

30. Hangody L, Rathonyi GK, Duska Z, et al. Autologous osteochondral mosaicplasty. Surgical technique. J Bone Joint Surg Am 2004;86-A(Suppl 1):65–72.

31. Camp CL, Stuart MJ, Krych AJ. Current concepts of articular cartilage restoration techniques in the knee. Sports Health 2014;6(3):265–73.

32. Brittberg M, Lindahl A, Nilsson A, et al. Treatment of deep cartilage defects in the knee with autologous chondrocyte transplantation. N Engl J Med 1994; 331(14):889–95.

33. Brittberg M. Autologous chondrocyte transplantation. Clin Orthop Relat Res 1999;(367 Suppl): S147–55.

34. McCarthy HS, Richardson JB, Parker JC, et al. Evaluating joint morbidity after chondral harvest for autologous chondrocyte implantation (ACI): a study of ACI-treated ankles and hips with a knee chondral harvest. Cartilage 2016;7(1):7–15.

35. Fu FH, Zurakowski D, Browne JE, et al. Autologous chondrocyte implantation versus debridement for treatment of full-thickness chondral defects of the knee: an observational cohort study with 3-year follow-up. Am J Sports Med 2005;33(11):1658–66.

36. Peterson L, Minas T, Brittberg M, et al. Two- to 9-year outcome after autologous chondrocyte transplantation of the knee. Clin Orthop Relat Res 2000;(374): 212–34.

37. Henderson I, Gui J, Lavigne P. Autologous chondrocyte implantation: natural history of postimplantation periosteal hypertrophy and effects of repair-site debridement on outcome. Arthroscopy 2006; 22(12):1318–1324 e1.

38. Henderson IJ, Tuy B, Connell D, et al. Prospective clinical study of autologous chondrocyte implantation and correlation with MRI at three and 12 months. J Bone Joint Surg Br 2003;85(7):1060–6.

39. Brown WE, Potter HG, Marx RG, et al. Magnetic resonance imaging appearance of cartilage repair in the knee. Clin Orthop Relat Res 2004;(422):214–23.

40. Kon E, Filardo G, Di Matteo B, et al. Matrix assisted autologous chondrocyte transplantation for cartilage treatment: A systematic review. Bone Joint Res 2013;2(2):18–25.

41. Schuette HB, Kraeutler MJ, McCarty EC. Matrix-assisted autologous chondrocyte transplantation in the knee: a systematic review of mid- to long-term clinical outcomes. Orthop J Sports Med 2017;5(6). 2325967117709250.

42. Hoffman JK, Geraghty S, Protzman NM. Articular cartilage repair using marrow stimulation augmented with a viable chondral allograft: 9-month postoperative histological evaluation. Case Rep Orthop 2015; 2015:617365.

43. Hirahara AM, Mueller KW Jr. BioCartilage: a new biomaterial to treat chondral lesions. Sports Med Arthrosc Rev 2015;23(3):143–8.

44. Choi YS, Potter HG, Chun TJ. MR imaging of cartilage repair in the knee and ankle. Radiographics 2008;28(4):1043–59.

45. Glaser C. New techniques for cartilage imaging: T2 relaxation time and diffusion-weighted MR imaging. Radiol Clin North Am 2005;43(4):641–653, vii.

46. Marlovits S, Singer P, Zeller P, et al. Magnetic resonance observation of cartilage repair tissue (MOCART) for the evaluation of autologous chondrocyte transplantation: determination of interobserver variability and correlation to clinical outcome after 2 years. Eur J Radiol 2006;57(1):16–23.

47. Marlovits S, Striessnig G, Resinger CT, et al. Definition of pertinent parameters for the evaluation of articular cartilage repair tissue with high-resolution magnetic resonance imaging. Eur J Radiol 2004; 52(3):310–9.

48. Schreiner MM, Raudner M, Marlovits S, et al. The MOCART (Magnetic Resonance Observation of Cartilage Repair Tissue) 2.0 Knee Score and Atlas. Cartilage 2019. https://doi.org/10.1177/1947603519865308. 1947603519865308.

49. Schreiner MM, Raudner M, Rohrich S, et al. Reliability of the MOCART (Magnetic Resonance Observation of Cartilage Repair Tissue) 2.0 knee score for different cartilage repair techniques-a retrospective observational study. Eur Radiol 2021;31(8):5734–45.

50. Roemer FW, Guermazi A, Trattnig S, et al. Whole joint MRI assessment of surgical cartilage repair of the knee: cartilage repair osteoarthritis knee score (CROAKS). Osteoarthritis Cartilage 2014;22(6): 779–99.

51. Guermazi A, Roemer FW, Alizai H, et al. State of the art: MR imaging after knee cartilage repair surgery. Radiology 2015;277(1):23–43.

52. Link TM, Mischung J, Wortler K, et al. Normal and pathological MR findings in osteochondral autografts with longitudinal follow-up. Eur Radiol 2006; 16(1):88–96.

53. Trattnig S, Ba-Ssalamah A, Pinker K, et al. Matrix-based autologous chondrocyte implantation for cartilage repair: noninvasive monitoring by high-resolution magnetic resonance imaging. Magn Reson Imaging 2005;23(7):779–87. https://doi.org/10.1016/j.mri.2005.04.010.

MR Imaging of the Knee Bursae and Bursal Pathology

Joao R.T. Vicentini, MD, Connie Y. Chang, MD*

KEYWORDS

- Knee • Bursa • Bursal anatomy • Bursitis • MR imaging

KEY POINTS

- Bursae are synovial-lined structures usually seen around joints, tendons, and bones, with the main functions of cushioning and friction reduction.
- The different knee bursae are usually not visible on imaging studies unless they are filled with fluid or other material, which could be reactive to an injury to the surrounding structures, or related to primary bursal pathology.
- Because of their position, the anterior and medial knee bursae are the most frequently involved in direct injuries to the knee or repetitive trauma.
- Chronic bursitis may have heterogeneous appearance on imaging, making it a common mimicker of a periarticular soft tissue mass.
- Primary bursal pathology usually shows resemblance with intra-articular processes, given the presence of synovial tissue lining the bursal spaces. Secondary bursal involvement, however, is more common and usually related to varying degrees of communication with the joint space.

INTRODUCTION

Bursae are structures with synovial lining commonly found around joints and regions prone to attrition, such as along tendons and osseous eminences. In the knee, the different bursae provide mechanical cushioning for structures around the joint capsule, including the many knee ligaments and tendons. These bursal spaces are usually collapsed and not seen on normal imaging studies. However, in the setting of injury to the bursa itself or to the surrounding structures in the knee, a reactive process leads to increased production of synovial fluid and distention of the bursal space, which can then be appreciated on different imaging modalities.[1,2]

Although less common, primary benign and malignant processes can also affect the knee bursae, some of which show similarities with intra-articular pathology, because of their synovial origin.[3] In daily practice, differentiation of the knee bursae from cystic lesions, soft tissue masses, or fluid collections is sometimes necessary, therefore knowledge of the normal bursal anatomy and common pathology is important to avoid unnecessary imaging or intervention.

IMAGING TECHNIQUE

Although different imaging modalities are used for visualization of the knee bursae, MR imaging is usually the method of choice because of high soft tissue contrast.[2] Additional advantages include the evaluation of associated findings, such as internal derangement of the knee, and lack of ionizing radiation. Fluid-sensitive sequences, such as T2-weighted sequences with fat suppression or short tau inversion recovery, are usually preferred for identification of bursae and cysts around the knee.[2,4] Proton-density

Division of Musculoskeletal Imaging and Intervention, Department of Radiology, Massachusetts General Hospital, 55 Fruit Street, Yawkey 6E, Boston, MA 02114, USA
* Corresponding author.
E-mail address: cychang@mgh.harvard.edu

Magn Reson Imaging Clin N Am 30 (2022) 241–260
https://doi.org/10.1016/j.mric.2021.11.005
1064-9689/22/© 2021 Elsevier Inc. All rights reserved.

sequences with or without fat suppression can also be helpful for evaluation of the knee anatomy, cartilage, and synovium. Gradient echo sequences are indicated for specific cases, usually when there is concern for presence of blood products, which show characteristic features on gradient echo imaging, such as blooming artifact.[3,4] Intravenous gadolinium-based contrast is usually not necessary for assessment of the knee bursae, but may be indicated for evaluation of soft tissue masses. It can also be used for evaluation of infection; however, isolated synovial enhancement is not specific for an infectious process, and may be present in healthy individuals.[3,5]

Ultrasound is a helpful screening method when MR imaging is not readily available, with studies showing sensitivity of approximately 87% for detection of bursal fluid in the knee when compared with MR imaging as the gold standard.[6] Ultrasound limitations include difficulty in evaluating the deep bursal spaces and assessing for communication with the joint space. Another potential pitfall is the interpretation of debris or thickened synovium as a solid lesion.[7] Computed tomography (CT) is rarely used for assessment of bursal pathology given limited utility for evaluation of soft tissue detail, and radiation. Because most bursae show attenuation similar to the surrounding musculature, differentiation may be difficult unless intravenous contrast shows synovial enhancement, which is rarely necessary. Radiographs are not indicated for evaluation of knee bursae as the primary imaging method, but are helpful for troubleshooting when there is a question of associated soft tissue mineralization, calcified mass, or loose bodies.[7]

NORMAL ANATOMY

Anatomic studies have shown that despite individual variability, the different bursal spaces in the knee show a consistent distribution among most people, which helps identifying them on imaging studies.[8–12] Dividing the knee bursae into separate groups allows for better understanding of their relationship with the joint capsule, and with surrounding ligaments and tendons.

The anterior knee bursae include the prepatellar, superficial infrapatellar, and deep infrapatellar bursae (**Fig. 1**). The suprapatellar recess is also included in this discussion because it develops embryologically as a bursa, and incomplete fusion with the knee joint can lead to additional pathology (discussed later). The medial knee bursae include the pes anserine bursa; medial collateral ligament (MCL) bursa; semimembranosus MCL (SM-MCL) bursa; and the bursa between the distal

semimembranosus tendon and the medial head of the gastrocnemius, which usually communicates with the joint space, leading to the formation of a Baker cyst (**Fig. 2**). The lateral knee bursae include the popliteus bursa; the lateral collateral ligament–biceps femoris bursa; the lateral collateral ligament–popliteus tendon bursa; and the iliotibial band bursa, which is considered an adventitious bursa, formed secondary to chronic friction (**Fig. 3**).

Most bursae do not communicate with the joint, except for the semimembranosus–medial gastrocnemius bursa, and some of them may show internal plicae, which are linear structures formed by folded synovial tissue, believed to be remnants of embryologic synovial membranes.[3] In the knee joint, four main plicae may be present: (1) the suprapatellar, (2) infrapatellar, (3) medial, and (4) lateral plicae.[13] When present, a plica is identified as a band of tissue with low signal on most MR imaging sequences.[3]

Anterior Knee

Suprapatellar recess
The suprapatellar recess develops as a separate synovial-lined space anterior to the distal femur and cranial to the knee joint, but in approximately 85% of people, the septum separating the bursa and the knee joint involutes during fetal development.[7,14,15] A residual suprapatellar plica may be present (**Fig. 4**).[16] In case of incomplete regression, an imperforate suprapatellar septum may lead to accumulation of fluid or thickened synovium in the original bursal space, which can mimic a soft tissue mass.[4,17]

Prepatellar bursa
Anatomic studies have demonstrated that the prepatellar bursa has three layers of tissue: (1) a superficial fascia, (2) an intermediate aponeurotic layer, and (3) deep dense fibers adherent to the quadriceps and patellar cortex, which create different combinations of bursal spaces.[8,18] On imaging studies, however, a bilaminar or trilaminar appearance is rarely seen.[7] Most commonly, a distended prepatellar bursa presents as a single fluid-filled saccular structure anterior to the patella (**Fig. 5**).

Deep infrapatellar bursa
The deep infrapatellar bursa is located between the distal third of the patellar tendon and the tibial tuberosity (**Fig. 6**). Anatomic studies have shown that a deep infrapatellar bursa is virtually always present.[9,19] However, studies using MR imaging in asymptomatic and symptomatic subjects have identified a deep infrapatellar bursa in 41% and

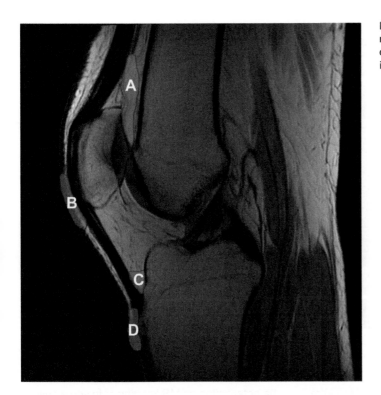

Fig. 1. Anterior knee bursae. (*A*) Suprapatellar (recess), (*B*) prepatellar, (*C*) deep infrapatellar, and (*D*) superficial infrapatellar.

68% of cases, respectively.[20,21] Association with Osgood-Schlatter has also been described, and decrease of bursal size after resolution of symptoms.[22] On MR imaging, the sagittal plane and fluid-sensitive sequences are usually preferred for a better evaluation of this bursa, given the small size and location.[21] Although communication with the joint space is present in some cases, a study evaluating 213 knee MR imaging examinations showed no correlation between presence of joint

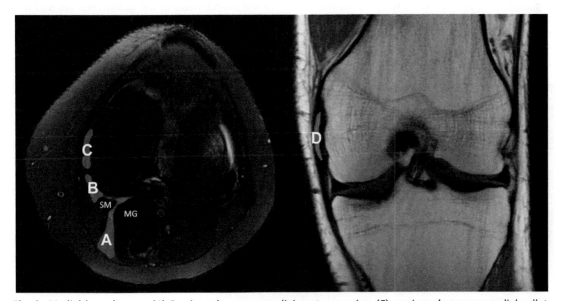

Fig. 2. Medial knee bursae. (*A*) Semimembranosus-medial gastrocnemius, (*B*) semimembranosus–medial collateral ligament, (*C*) pes anserine, and (*D*) medial collateral ligament. MG, medial head of the gastrocnemius; SM, semimembranosus.

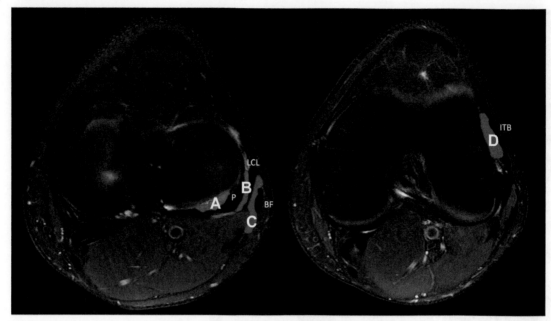

Fig. 3. Lateral knee bursae. (*A*) Popliteus bursa, (*B*) lateral collateral ligament–popliteus (LCL-P) bursa, (*C*) lateral collateral ligament–biceps femoris (LCL-BF) bursa, and (*D*) iliotibial band (ITB) bursa.

effusion and the presence or size of a deep infra-patellar bursa.[21]

Superficial infrapatellar bursa

The superficial infrapatellar bursa is located between the tibial tuberosity and the pretibial subcutaneous tissues, anterior to the patellar tendon (**Fig. 7**). Anatomic studies have failed to identify this bursal space in many of the specimens, which suggests it may not be always present.[20,23] Although the presence of an internal septation has been described, the superficial infrapatellar bursa is usually too small for detailed

characterization on MR imaging.[23] In some cases, such as in the setting of trauma, this bursa may be difficult to identify because of surrounding edema of the adjacent pretibial soft tissues.[7]

Medial Knee

Semimembranosus–medial gastrocnemius

Distention of the bursa located between the origin of the medial head of the gastrocnemius and the distal semimembranosus tendon leads to the formation of a Baker cyst, the most commonly seen cystic structure about the knee, and first described

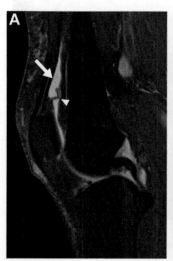
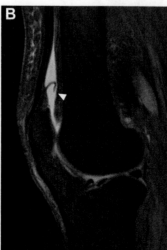

Fig. 4. (*A*) Sagittal T2-weighted sequence with fat suppression (T2FS) image shows fluid in the suprapatellar recess (*arrow*) with a suprapatellar plica (*arrowhead*). (*B*) As seen in most people, the suprapatellar plica (*arrowhead*) is not complete, which results in communication between the primitive suprapatellar bursa and the joint space.

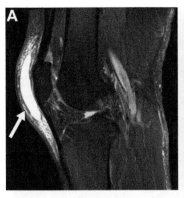
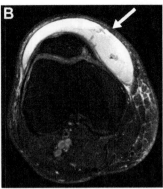

Fig. 5. A 63-year-old man with anterior knee soft tissue swelling. Sagittal (*A*) and axial (*B*) T2FS images show a distended prepatellar bursa (*arrows*) with surrounding edema.

by William M. Baker in 1877.[10,24] This bursa shows communication with the joint space in up to 50% of people, which is one of the reasons why Baker cysts are a common finding, present in 5% to 38% of adult knee MR imaging studies.[25–28] Baker cysts are less common in children, with a prevalence of 6.3% in one case series with 393 pediatric knee MR imaging studies.[11] A possible explanation for the lower prevalence in younger patients is the association of Baker cyst with pathology less frequent in this age group, such as osteoarthritis and different types of internal derangement of the knee.[25] Baker cysts may rupture and dissect through the adjacent fascial planes, which is usually associated with pain, mimicking other pathologies, such as venous thrombosis (**Fig. 8**).[28]

Pes anserine bursa

The pes anserine bursa is the most superficial bursa of the medial knee, located between the tibial attachment of the MCL and the distal portion of the conjoined tendon formed by the sartorius, gracilis, and semitendinosus (**Fig. 9**).[2] Studies using MR imaging have shown a prevalence of pes anserine bursal distention of up to 2.5% among symptomatic patients, and up to 5.0% in asymptomatic patients, which suggests that presence of fluid on MR imaging is not enough for the diagnosis of bursitis, and additional findings, such as surrounding edema or synovitis, may be necessary for the diagnosis.[20,29] Clinically, conditions affecting the pes anserine bursa may mimic injuries of other medial knee structures, such as the medial meniscus or MCL; therefore, MR imaging is usually indicated for proper diagnosis.[30] Pes anserine bursitis is usually associated with chronic overuse, and it is often seen in runners.[28]

Semimembranosus–medial collateral ligament bursa

The SM-MCL bursa is a small bursal space located superior and posterior to the pes anserine bursa, protecting the semimembranosus tendon from friction against the static MCL and proximal tibia (**Fig. 10**). This bursa wraps around the distal semimembranosus tendon and may show an inverted U-shaped appearance when distended.[31] Clinically, patients with SM-MCL bursitis usually

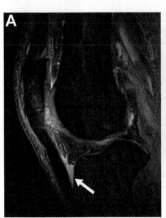
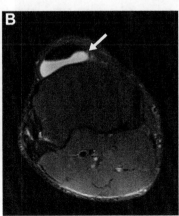

Fig. 6. A 33-year-old man with prior traumatic injury to the proximal patellar tendon. Sagittal (*A*) and axial (*B*) T2FS images show fluid in the deep infrapatellar bursa (*arrows*), between the distal patellar tendon and the proximal tibia.

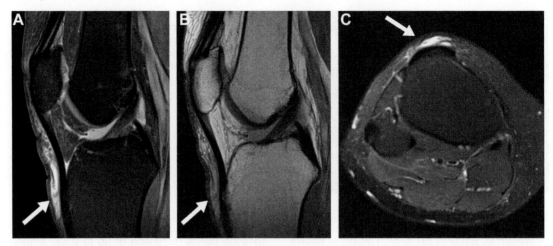

Fig. 7. A 45-year-old woman with painless swelling anterior to the tibial tuberosity. Sagittal T2FS (*A*) and proton density (*B*) images, and axial T2FS (*C*) image show distention of the superficial infrapatellar bursa (*arrows*) anterior to the distal patellar tendon.

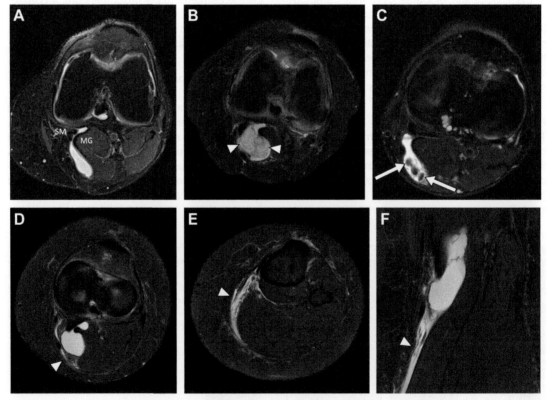

Fig. 8. Axial (*A-E*) and coronal (*F*) T2FS images of different patients showing possible appearances of a Baker cyst. (*A*) The most common presentation is a simple fluid-filled cystic structure between the SM and MG. (*B*) When there is associated synovitis, synovial thickening or internal septations can be seen (*arrowheads*). (*C*) Because of the Baker cyst position, loose bodies can usually be seen in the dependent portions of the cyst (*arrows*). (*D-F*) Partially ruptured Baker cyst with fluid tracking down along the fascial planes in the lower leg (*arrowheads*).

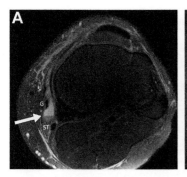
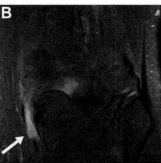

Fig. 9. A 60-year-old man with progressive pain in the medial left knee when walking. Axial (*A*) and coronal (*B*) T2FS images showing distention of the pes anserine bursa with fluid-fluid levels (*arrows*), deep to the distal aspect of the tendons in the medial knee. G, gracilis; S, sartorius; ST, semitendinosus tendon.

present with posteromedial knee pain.[7] Distinguishing this bursa from the pes anserine bursa or from small amount of fluid in the semimembranosus–medial gastrocnemius bursa may be difficult; however, these bursal spaces usually do not communicate.[31] Another potential pitfall is a posteromedial parameniscal cyst, which is differentiated by finding an associated meniscal tear.[2]

Medial collateral ligament bursa

The structures supporting the medial knee capsule are divided into three layers. The most superficial one is the crural fascia, followed by the superficial portion of the MCL or tibial collateral ligament, and finally the deep portion of the MCL blended with the joint capsule itself.[11] The medial or tibial collateral ligament bursa is located between the deep and superficial fibers of the MCL.[11,32] The distended bursa usually shows an elongated configuration, between both components of the ligament on the axial plane (**Fig. 11**). Although isolated MCL bursal distention is an uncommon MR imaging finding, anatomic studies have demonstrated that this bursa is present in approximately 90% of cases.[11,32] Similar to the other bursae, it can only be identified on MR imaging when it is filled with fluid, usually in the setting of inflammation or traumatic injury of the medial knee structures.[11]

In these situations, differentiation from a medial parameniscal cyst may also be necessary.[2]

Lateral Knee

The lateral knee bursae show higher individual variability when compared with the medial and anterior knee. The most consistently seen lateral knee bursae include the lateral collateral ligament–biceps femoris bursa; lateral collateral ligament–popliteus tendon bursa; and the popliteal bursa, which is located deep to the popliteus tendon (**Figs. 12 and 13**).[3,12] The popliteal bursa may also show communication with the proximal tibiofibular joint.[7] Some authors also include a recess located between the lateral head of the gastrocnemius and the joint capsule among the different knee bursae, but this region is usually contiguous with the joint space, forming a recess rather than a separate bursa.[3]

Located between the distal aspect of the iliotibial band and the lateral femoral condyle and proximal tibia above the Gerdy tubercle, the iliotibial bursa is not considered a true bursa by most authors, but rather a secondary or adventitious bursa, formed in the setting of chronic friction or overuse (**Fig. 14**).[2,3] Typically seen in long-distance runners, the findings of edema and adventitious bursa formation deep to the iliotibial

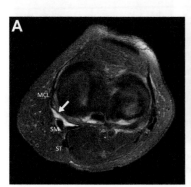
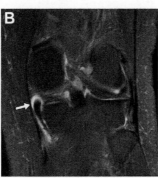

Fig. 10. A 59-year-old woman with right knee pain when running. Axial (*A*) and coronal (*B*) T2FS images show a fluid-filled semimembranosus–medial collateral ligament bursa (*arrows*).

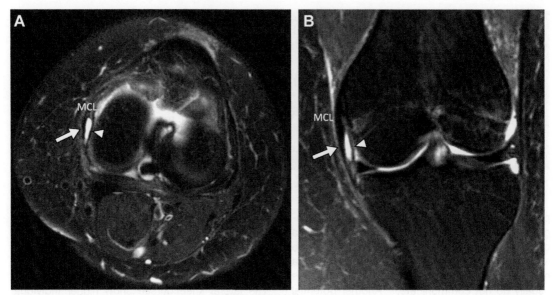

Fig. 11. Axial (*A*) and coronal (*B*) T2FS images show distention of the MCL bursa, between the superficial (*arrow*) and deep (*arrowhead*) ligament fibers.

band is usually termed iliotibial band friction syndrome.[33]

BURSAL PATHOLOGY
Bursitis

Multiple different processes may lead to inflammation of the bursal synovial lining, resulting in increased production of synovial fluid and subsequent bursal distention, which is generically referred to as bursitis.[3] In many cases, bursitis may be reactive to an injury involving an adjacent structure, such as a ligament or tendon. When the bursa is primarily affected, the most common causes include acute or repetitive trauma, chronic overuse, infection, and inflammatory

arthropathy.[1–3,7,28] Chronic repetitive trauma is the most common cause of anterior knee bursitis, classically described in patients with history of occupational kneeling, such as housemaid's knee (prepatellar bursitis) or clergyman's knee (superficial infrapatellar bursitis).[28,34]

Acute direct or indirect trauma to the knee may cause bleeding into a bursal space. On MR imaging, hemorrhagic bursitis may show layering of different fluid components during the acute phase, but over time the appearance becomes more heterogeneous, with areas of low signal related to evolving blood products, especially when imaging is performed days or weeks after the traumatic event.[3] Blood products may show increased T1 signal, which is helpful for diagnosis (**Fig. 15**).

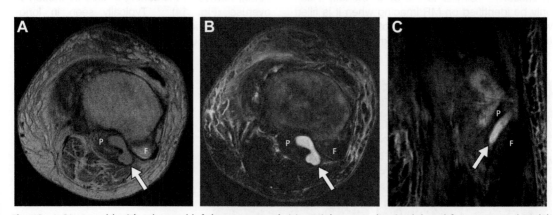

Fig. 12. A 61 year old with advanced left knee osteoarthritis. Axial proton-density (*A*) and fat-suppressed T2 (*B*) images show fluid-filled bursa along the popliteus tendon (*arrows*). (*C*) Coronal T2FS image shows the distended bursa between the popliteus tendon (P) and the fibular head (F).

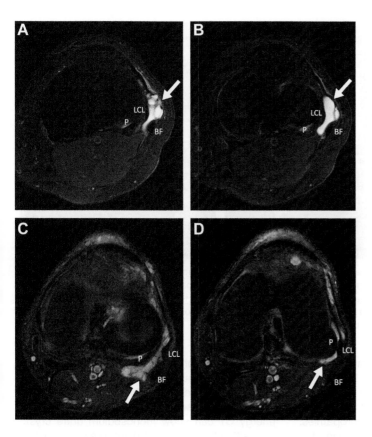

Fig. 13. A 62-year-old woman with lateral knee swelling. (*A-D*) Axial T2FS images show fluid distention and septations within the lateral collateral ligament–biceps femoris bursa (*arrows* in *A* and *B*), and lateral collateral ligament–popliteus bursa (*arrows* in *C* and *D*). BF, biceps femoris; LCL, lateral collateral ligament; P, popliteus tendon.

Chronic solid-appearing or partially calcified areas within an organizing hematoma may be erroneously interpreted as a soft tissue mass.[35] A differential for hemorrhagic prepatellar bursitis is a degloving injury or Morel-Lavallée lesion, which results from a shearing mechanism at the interface between the deep subcutaneous tissues and the anterior prepatellar fascia (**Fig. 16**).[4] Some distinguishing features of a prepatellar Morel-Lavallée lesion include large dimensions, location slightly eccentric to the patella, and presence of fat lobules within the hemorrhagic collection.[4]

Inflammation and Infection

The knee joint is affected by many different inflammatory conditions, including rheumatoid arthritis and crystalline arthropathies, such as gout and calcium pyrophosphate dehydrate arthropathy.[3] Although intra-articular involvement is the

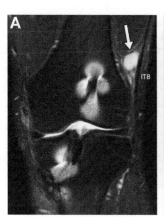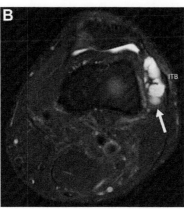

Fig. 14. A 28-year-old male runner with previous anterior cruciate ligament reconstruction. Coronal (*A*) and axial (*B*) T2FS images show a loculated cystic structure between the distal ITB and the lateral femoral condyle, consistent with adventitious bursa formation (*arrow*).

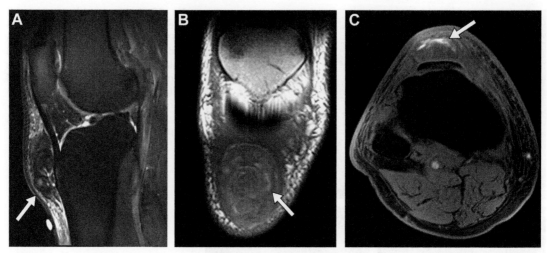

Fig. 15. A 56-year-old man on anticoagulation therapy presented with question of anterior knee soft tissue mass. (*A*) Sagittal T2FS image shows low signal material within the superficial infrapatellar bursa (*arrow*). (*B*) Coronal T1 image shows areas with increased T1 signal associated with this finding (*arrow*). (*C*) Axial fat-suppressed T1 image shows persistent high signal in the superficial infrapatellar bursa (*arrow*), consistent with hemorrhagic bursitis. Clinical follow-up showed eventual resolution of these findings.

predominant manifestation of inflammatory arthropathies, different bursae can also be affected because of the presence of synovial tissue and eventual communication with the joint space.[3,4]

Among the different inflammatory arthropathies, gout is one of the most commonly involving the knee.[36] In the acute setting, a gout flare may be similar to any other inflammatory arthropathy, with enhancing synovitis and surrounding edema. Over time, deposition of monosodium urate crystals leads to the formation of extra-articular tophi, most commonly seen along the popliteus tendon, popliteal notch in the lateral femoral condyle, patellar tendon, and distal quadriceps.[36,37] Bursal involvement is variable, and more common for the prepatellar bursa, possibly because of the proximity with the extensor apparatus and frequent

deposition of tophi in the anterior knee soft tissues (**Fig. 17**).[36,37] Gouty tophi usually show low signal on T1 images and variable signal intensity on fluid-sensitive sequences (**Fig. 18**).[3,37] Dual-energy CT can show monosodium urate crystal deposition to support the diagnosis (**Fig. 19**).[38]

Bursal inflammation may also be secondary to an underlying infection. Septic bursitis usually results from traumatic injury and inoculation of an infectious agent into the skin with further translocation into the bursal space (**Fig. 20**).[39,40] In the knee, the prepatellar bursa is most commonly affected, and the main infectious agent is *Staphylococcus aureus*.[39–41] MR imaging findings associated with septic bursitis include bursal distention, wall thickening, enhancing synovitis, and complex fluid with debris, although these

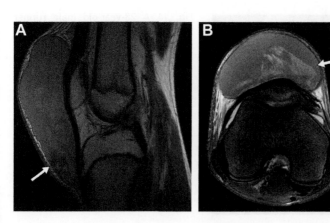

Fig. 16. A 17-year-old boy with history hemophilia and injury of the right knee while wrestling. Sagittal (*A*) and axial fat-suppressed (*B*) proton density images show large fluid collection with heterogeneous material anterior to the patella, distal quadriceps, and patellar tendon (*arrows*). Despite the location typical for prepatellar hemorrhagic bursitis, the size of the hematoma is suggestive of a degloving injury (Morel-Lavallée).

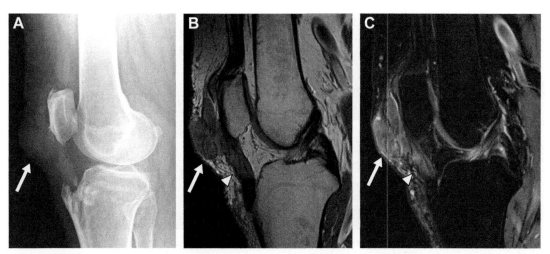

Fig. 17. A 68-year-old man with biopsy-proven gout. (*A*) Radiograph shows marked prepatellar soft tissue swelling (*arrow*) and patellar tendon thickening. Sagittal proton density (*B*) and T2FS (*C*) images show soft tissue tophi involving the prepatellar bursa (*arrows*) and the patellar tendon (*arrowheads*).

features are not specific for infection and could be seen with other etiologies.[42] If present, soft tissue gas is seen as foci of signal void.[42] Antibiotic therapy is the main line of treatment, and surgery is reserved for recurrent or refractory cases.[39]

Tumors and Pseudotumors

Synovial chondromatosis

Primary synovial chondromatosis is a benign entity in which hyaline cartilaginous bodies are formed within the synovium with progressive enlargement

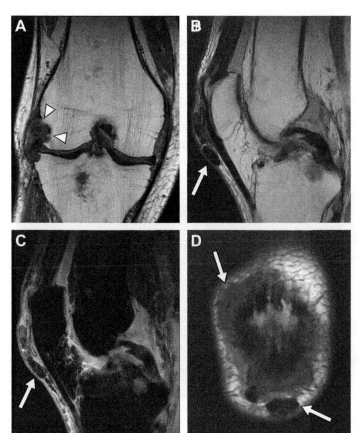

Fig. 18. A 69-year-old male patient with known gout. (*A*) Coronal T1 image shows bone erosions involving the popliteal groove at the lateral femoral condyle (*arrowheads*) with diffuse popliteal tendon thickening, a typical finding for gout in the knee. Sagittal proton density (*B*) and T2FS (*C*), and coronal T1 (*D*) images show low signal tophi involving the prepatellar bursa (*arrows*).

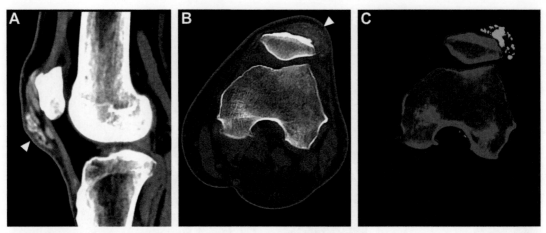

Fig. 19. Dual-energy CT for gout. Sagittal (*A*) and axial (*B*) CT images show calcified tophi involving the prepatellar bursa (*arrowheads*). (*C*) Reformatted color-coded image shows evidence of monosodium urate crystal deposition (*green*), confirming the diagnosis of gout.

and eventual detachment from the synovial lining.[43] Males are affected two to four times more frequently than females.[43] Primary synovial chondromatosis affects primarily large joints, but the synovial tissue in a bursa or tendon sheath can also be involved.[44–49] Synovial chondromatosis within a bursa or tendon sheath most commonly presents as a slowly enlarging mass with or without associated pain.[44] Although bursal and tenosynovial involvement has been reported mostly in the upper extremities, involvement of isolated bursal spaces around the knee, such as the pes anserine bursa or a suprapatellar bursa with an imperforate suprapatellar plica, has also been reported (**Fig. 21**).[48,49]

Secondary synovial chondromatosis occurs when the cartilaginous and osteocartilaginous bodies are formed during shedding of the articular cartilage in the setting of degenerative joint disease. Because of high prevalence of knee osteoarthritis, secondary synovial chondromatosis is much more common than its primary counterpart.[3] In this scenario, however, loose bodies are only seen in a bursa if there is communication with the joint space (**Fig. 22**). For that reason, the most common locations for loose bodies in the knee are the suprapatellar recess and within a Baker cyst. Bursal synovial chondromatosis has also been described following the resection of an adjacent osteochondroma.[48,50]

Initially, the cartilaginous bodies are better seen on MR imaging, with low signal on T1- and T2-weighted images. Over time, these cartilaginous bodies undergo progressive calcification, making

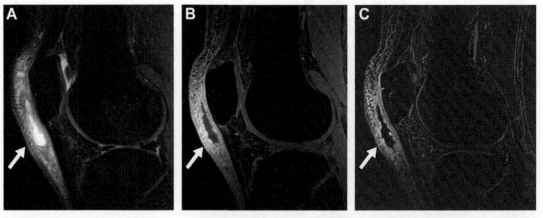

Fig. 20. A 21-year-old landscaper presenting with anterior knee swelling, pain, and erythema. Sagittal T2FS (*A*), postcontrast fat-suppressed T1 (*B*), and subtraction (*C*) images show distended prepatellar bursa with enhancing thickened synovium, and surrounding edema, consistent with septic prepatellar bursitis (*arrows*).

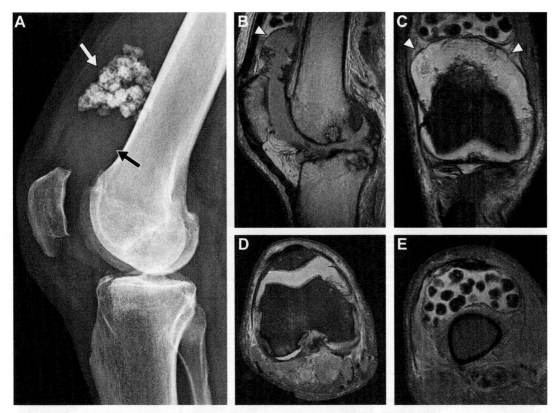

Fig. 21. A 74-year-old man with left knee swelling. (*A*) Multiple partially calcified bodies project over the supra-patellar region (*white arrow*). Soft tissue density is also seen more inferiorly (*black arrow*). (*B-E*) Fat-suppressed proton density images show a complete suprapatellar plica (*arrowheads*) with multiple loose bodies in a supra-patellar bursa, separate from the effusion and synovitis seen more inferiorly in the joint space.

them easily identifiable on radiographs or CT.[44] Endochondral ossification may also occur, leading to MR imaging signal similar to normal bone marrow.[3]

Tenosynovial giant cell tumor

Tenosynovial giant cell tumor is a term used in the most recent World Health Organization classification to group different conditions characterized by

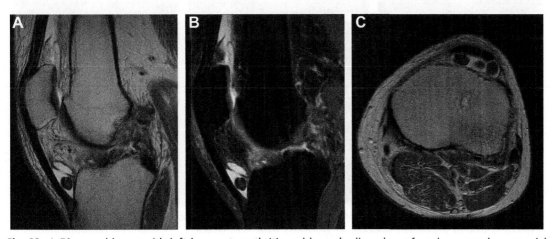

Fig. 22. A 50-year-old man with left knee osteoarthritis and loose bodies, also referred as secondary synovial chondromatosis. Presence of loose bodies in the infrapatellar bursa is suggestive of communication with the joint space.

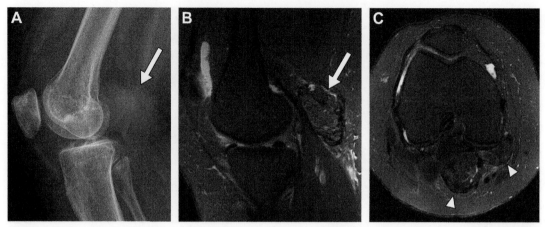

Fig. 23. A 51-year-old woman with tenosynovial giant cell tumor, diffuse type (formerly known as pigmented villonodular synovitis). (*A*) Right knee radiograph shows area of increased density projecting over the popliteal fossa (*arrow*). Sagittal (*B*) and axial (*C*) T2FS images show masslike soft tissue thickening with predominantly low T2 signal filling up a Baker cyst (*arrows*). The presence of hemosiderin leads to the typical low signal on most MR imaging sequences.

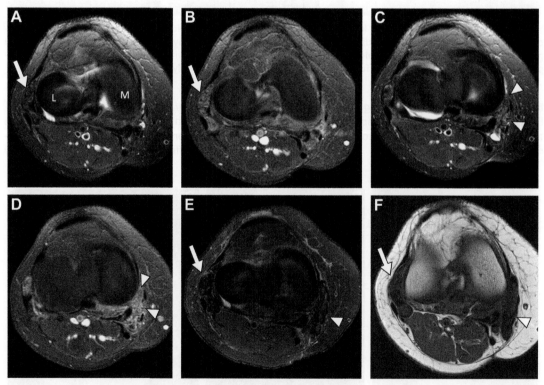

Fig. 24. A 61-year-old woman with a long history of right knee tenosynovial giant cell tumor, diffuse type (formerly known as pigmented villonodular synovitis). Axial T2FS (*A* and *C*), postcontrast fat-suppressed T1 (*B* and *D*), and follow-up T2FS (*E*) and T1 (*F*) images show enhancing soft tissue with low T2 and T1 signal involving the lateral and medial knee bursae, including the LCL-biceps femoris bursa (*arrows*) and semimembranosus-MCL bursa (*arrowheads*). L, lateral femoral condyle; M, medial femoral condyle.

hypertrophic proliferation of the synovium with osteoclast-like, multinucleated giant cells, usually involving joints, tendon sheaths, or bursae.[51,52] The localized type is also known as giant cell tumor of the tendon sheath or focal nodular synovitis, and usually presents as a soft tissue nodule or mass, most frequently associated with the tendons in the hands.[52,53] The diffuse type, formerly known as pigmented villonodular synovitis, usually involves large joints, with the knee being most commonly affected, and representing up to 80% of the cases.[53,54] During the course of the disease, a typical feature is the accumulation of hemosiderin-laden macrophage deposits, which leads to the characteristic findings of a thickened synovium with low signal on T1- and T2-weighted images.[3] The iron within the hemosiderin deposits results in a form of susceptibility artifact called blooming artifact, characterized by markedly low signal on gradient echo sequences.[54] When the lesion is intra-articular, bone erosions are commonly seen, which are believed to result from a combination of increased intra-articular pressure from the thickened synovium, and

proteolytic enzymes produced by the giant cells.[53,54] For having a larger joint space, the knee shows a prevalence of bone erosions of approximately 25%, versus up to 90% for other large joints with smaller joint spaces, such as the hip and shoulder.[54] Bursal involvement by diffuse tenosynovial giant cell tumor in the knee is most commonly seen because of secondary extension of lesions originated in the joint space, although rare cases of isolated bursal involvement have also been reported, such as in the pes anserine bursa (**Figs. 23 and 24**).[55–58]

Lipoma arborescens

Lipoma arborescens is a rare synovial condition where the subsynovial tissue is replaced by mature adipose cells.[3] Also called villous lipomatous proliferation of the synovial membrane, this entity is favored to be a benign reaction to a chronic underlying process, such as osteoarthritis and rheumatoid arthritis.[59] Similar to other synovial conditions, lipoma arborescens is most commonly seen in joints, although bursal and tenosynovial involvement seems to be more

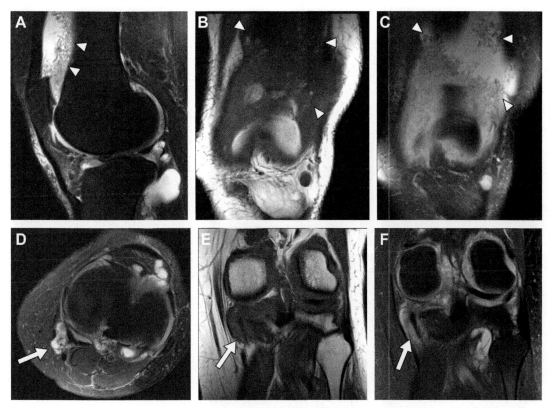

Fig. 25. A 56-year-old woman with seronegative oligoarticular inflammatory arthritis. Sagittal T2FS (*A*), and coronal T1 (*B*) and T2FS (*C*) images of the left knee show frond-like synovitis with fatty signal on T1, consistent with lipoma arborescens (*arrowheads*). (*D-F*) Additional images show similar-appearing finding in the pes anserine bursa, which may reflect communication with the joint space or separate bursal inflammation (*arrows*).

frequent in the upper extremities, notably in the bicipitoradial bursa.[60–65] Only two cases of isolated, extra-articular bursal involvement in the knee have been reported, one of them in the iliotibial band bursal space, and the other one described as involving a lateral knee bursae, not further specified.[66,67] On MR imaging, typical features for lipoma arborescens include synovitis with a frond-like appearance and T1 signal similar to the subcutaneous fat, usually without significant postcontrast enhancement (**Fig. 25**).[3,60]

Synovial sarcoma

Musculoskeletal synovial sarcomas usually originate in the extremities, with a high prevalence in the knee region.[68] Despite the name, synovial sarcomas do not originate from synovial tissue and an intra-articular origin is extremely rare, accounting for approximately 5% of the cases.[68,69] There are three main histologic subtypes based on the proportion of mesenchymal and epithelial differentiation: (1) monophasic (50%–60%), (2) biphasic (20%–30%), and (3) poorly differentiated (15%–25%).[70]

Synovial sarcomas in the knee usually originate in a juxta-articular position. Intra-articular involvement is most commonly related to joint invasion by an adjacent mass.[69] Because these lesions originate in the soft tissues around the knee joint, involvement of the different knee bursae may also occur (**Fig. 26**). Primary bursal origin also seems to be rare, with only one case involving the knee reported in literature, which was described as a lesion arising in a bursal space associated with the semimembranosus tendon.[71]

PITFALLS

Evaluation of cystic-appearing structures in the knee should include assessment of communication with the joint space. When there is large joint effusion, the distended joint recesses may extend along ligaments and tendons, simulating bursal spaces.[1,2] Ganglion and synovial cysts are also common mimickers.[3,28] By definition, ganglion cysts are also noncommunicating, and is usually differentiated from distended bursal spaces based on the location and anatomic landmarks. Parameniscal cysts are differentiated by identifying an underlying meniscal tear. Standard knee MR imaging protocols are usually enough for characterization of the different knee bursae. If necessary, knee arthrogram with or without subsequent MR imaging can also be considered for differentiation of noncommunicating bursae from prominent joint recesses.[7]

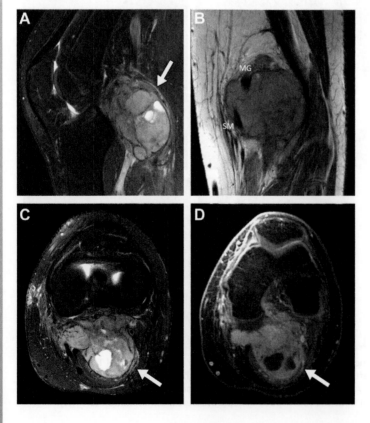

Fig. 26. An 18-year-old man with a posterior left knee synovial sarcoma. (*A*) Sagittal T2FS image shows a large, heterogeneous mass in the popliteal fossa (*arrow*). (*B*) Coronal T1 image shows that a component of the mass (*arrow*) insinuates between the SM and MG. Axial T2FS (*C*) and contrast-enhanced fat-suppressed T1 (*D*) images show that despite being centered at the midline, the mass (*arrow*) also involves the SM-GM bursa and posterior joint capsule. Central nonenhancing areas are likely related to necrosis.

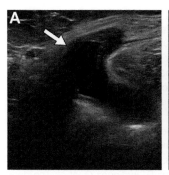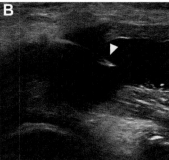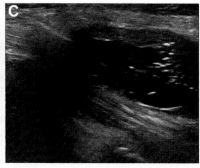

Fig. 27. Ultrasound-guided aspiration and corticosteroid injection into a Baker cyst. (*A*) Transverse image of the medial aspect of the popliteal fossa shows the typical comma-shaped appearance of a Baker cyst between the semimembranosus and medial head of the gastrocnemius (*arrow*). (*B*) Aspiration is performed under ultrasound guidance after the needle tip (*arrowhead*) advanced into the cyst. (*C*) Injected corticosteroid and tiny foci of air are seen as hyperechoic foci within the cyst.

Chronic bursitis may show heterogeneous appearance on MR imaging, with low signal on T1- and T2-weighted images, and variable synovial enhancement, mimicking a solid soft tissue mass.[72] Follow-up imaging or eventually imaging-guided biopsy may be needed for a definitive diagnosis.

INTERVENTION

Symptomatic patients may benefit from bursal aspiration to alleviate bursal distention. Ultrasound guidance is preferred because of widespread availability, lack of ionizing radiation, and easy visualization of distended bursae caused by the presence of fluid.[6] Aspiration can usually be performed in an outpatient setting with local anesthesia, and, if indicated, corticosteroids can also be administered during the same procedure.[73] This is frequently performed for Baker cysts (**Fig. 27**).[74]

Imaging-guided aspiration can also be part of the diagnostic work-up for septic bursitis. Samples are sent for cell count and cultures to assist with further treatment planning.[39] Ultrasound-guided synovial biopsy can also be performed if there is little bursal fluid. Because of overlap of clinical and imaging findings with other causes of bursal inflammation, such as crystalline arthropathies, additional testing for crystals is also recommended. In this scenario, corticosteroid injection is usually avoided until obtaining the aspiration results, because of the potential of transitory immunosuppression and risk of worsening an underlying infection.

SUMMARY

The different knee bursae exert an important function counterbalancing external forces and cushioning the joint capsule and surrounding ligaments and tendons. MR imaging with fluid-sensitive sequences is the best imaging choice for adequate characterization of bursal anatomy, and differentiation from periarticular cysts and fluid collections. It is also important to remember that bursal pathology may resemble, or be accompanied by intra-articular processes because of the presence of synovial lining and eventual communication with the joint space.

CLINICS CARE POINTS

- Chronic hemorrhagic bursitis may mimic a solid mass on MR imaging. Because bursal anatomy is consistent among most individuals, a solid-appearing lesion in a location typical for a knee bursa may benefit from short-term follow-up before recommending an invasive procedure.

- Septic bursitis is most commonly seen in the anterior knee, usually resulting from penetrating trauma. In the appropriate clinical setting, presence of marked synovitis, postcontrast enhancement, and surrounding edema should raise concern for this etiology.

- Imaging-guided aspiration and corticosteroid injection is performed for treatment of bursal-related symptoms, usually under ultrasound guidance. In cases of infection, diagnostic aspiration can also be performed to assist with treatment planning.

DISCLOSURES

The authors have nothing to disclose.

REFERENCES

1. Janzen DL, Peterfy CG, Forbes JR, et al. Cystic lesions around the knee joint: MR imaging findings. AJR Am J Roentgenol 1994;163(1):155–61.
2. McCarthy CL, McNally EG. The MRI appearance of cystic lesions around the knee. Skeletal Radiol 2004; 33(4):187–209.
3. Chung CB, Boucher R, Resnick D. MR imaging of synovial disorders of the knee. Semin Musculoskelet Radiol 2009;13(4):303–25.
4. Flores DV, Mejía Gómez C, Pathria MN. Layered approach to the anterior knee: normal anatomy and disorders associated with anterior knee pain. Radiogr Rev Publ Radiol Soc N Am Inc 2018;38(7): 2069–101.
5. Boegård T, Johansson A, Rudling O, et al. Gadolinium-DTPA-enhanced MR imaging in asymptomatic knees. Acta Radiol Stockh Swed 1987 1996;37(6):877–82.
6. Draghi F, Corti R, Urciuoli L, et al. Knee bursitis: a sonographic evaluation. J Ultrasound 2015;18(3): 251–7.
7. Steinbach LS, Stevens KJ. Imaging of cysts and bursae about the knee. Radiol Clin North Am 2013; 51(3):433–54.
8. Aguiar RO, Viegas FC, Fernandez RY, et al. The prepatellar bursa: cadaveric investigation of regional anatomy with MRI after sonographically guided bursography. AJR Am J Roentgenol 2007;188(4):W355–8.
9. LaPrade RF. The anatomy of the deep infrapatellar bursa of the knee. Am J Sports Med 1998;26(1):129–32.
10. Lindgren PG. Gastrocnemio-semimembranosus bursa and its relation to the knee joint. II. Post mortem radiography. Acta Radiol Diagn (Stockh) 1977; 18(6):698–704.
11. De Maeseneer M, Shahabpour M, Van Roy F, et al. MR imaging of the medial collateral ligament bursa: findings in patients and anatomic data derived from cadavers. AJR Am J Roentgenol 2001;177(4):911–7.
12. LaPrade RF, Hamilton CD. The fibular collateral ligament-biceps femoris bursa. An anatomic study. Am J Sports Med 1997;25(4):439–43.
13. Kim S-J, Choe W-S. Arthroscopic findings of the synovial plicae of the knee. Arthrosc J Arthrosc Relat Surg 1997;13(1):33–41.
14. Zidorn T. Classification of the suprapatellar septum considering ontogenetic development. Arthrosc J Arthrosc Relat Surg 1992;8(4):459–64.
15. Deutsch AL, Resnick D, Dalinka MK, et al. Synovial plicae of the knee. Radiology 1981;141(3):627–34.
16. Yamamoto T, Akisue T, Marui T, et al. Isolated suprapatellar bursitis: computed tomographic and arthroscopic findings. Arthrosc J Arthrosc Relat Surg 2003;19(2):E10.
17. Ehlinger M, Moser T, Adam P, et al. Complete suprapatellar plica presenting like a tumor. Orthop Traumatol Surg Res OTSR 2009;95(6):447–50.
18. Dye SF, Campagna-Pinto D, Dye CC, et al. Soft-tissue anatomy anterior to the human patella. J Bone Joint Surg Am 2003;85(6):1012–7.
19. Klein W. Endoscopy of the deep infrapatellar bursa. Arthrosc J Arthrosc Relat Surg 1996;12(1):127–31.
20. Tschirch FTC, Schmid MR, Pfirrmann CWA, et al. Prevalence and size of meniscal cysts, ganglionic cysts, synovial cysts of the popliteal space, fluid-filled bursae, and other fluid collections in asymptomatic knees on MR imaging. AJR Am J Roentgenol 2003;180(5):1431–6.
21. Aydingoz U, Oguz B, Aydingoz O, et al. The deep infrapatellar bursa: prevalence and morphology on routine magnetic resonance imaging of the knee. J Comput Assist Tomogr 2004;28(4):557–61.
22. Rosenberg ZS, Kawelblum M, Cheung YY, et al. Osgood-Schlatter lesion: fracture or tendinitis? Scintigraphic, CT, and MR imaging features. Radiology 1992;185(3):853–8.
23. Viegas FC, Aguiar ROC, Gasparetto E, et al. Deep and superficial infrapatellar bursae: cadaveric investigation of regional anatomy using magnetic resonance after ultrasound-guided bursography. Skeletal Radiol 2007;36(1):41–6.
24. Baker WM. On the formation of synovial cysts in the leg in connection with disease of the knee-joint. 1877. Clin Orthop 1994;(299):2–10.
25. Miller TT, Staron RB, Koenigsberg T, et al. MR imaging of Baker cysts: association with internal derangement, effusion, and degenerative arthropathy. Radiology 1996;201(1):247–50.
26. Fielding JR, Franklin PD, Kustan J. Popliteal cysts: a reassessment using magnetic resonance imaging. Skeletal Radiol 1991;20(6):433–5.
27. Martí-Bonmatí L, Mollá E, Dosdá R, et al. MR imaging of Baker cysts: prevalence and relation to internal derangements of the knee. Magma N Y N 2000;10(3):205–10.
28. Beaman FD, Peterson JJ. MR imaging of cysts, ganglia, and bursae about the knee. Radiol Clin North Am 2007;45(6):969–82.
29. Rennie WJ, Saifuddin A. Pes anserine bursitis: incidence in symptomatic knees and clinical presentation. Skeletal Radiol 2005;34(7):395–8.
30. Forbes JR, Helms CA, Janzen DL. Acute pes anserine bursitis: MR imaging. Radiology 1995;194(2):525–7.
31. Rothstein CP, Laorr A, Helms CA, et al. Semimembranosus-tibial collateral ligament bursitis: MR imaging findings. Am J Roentgenol 1996;166(4):875–7.
32. Lee JK, Yao L. Tibial collateral ligament bursa: MR imaging. Radiology 1991;178(3):855–7.
33. Murphy BJ, Hechtman KS, Uribe JW, et al. Iliotibial band friction syndrome: MR imaging findings. Radiology 1992;185(2):569–71.
34. Marra MD, Crema MD, Chung M, et al. MRI features of cystic lesions around the knee. Knee 2008;15(6): 423–38.

35. Stahnke M, Mangham DC, Davies AM. Calcific hae-morrhagic bursitis anterior to the knee mimicking a soft tissue sarcoma: report of two cases. Skeletal Radiol 2004;33(6):363–6.

36. Ko K-H, Hsu Y-C, Lee H-S, et al. Tophaceous gout of the knee: revisiting MRI patterns in 30 patients. J Clin Rheumatol Pract Rep Rheum Musculoskelet Dis 2010;16(5):209–14.

37. Yu JS, Chung C, Recht M, et al. MR imaging of to-phaceous gout. AJR Am J Roentgenol 1997; 168(2):523–7.

38. Desai MA, Peterson JJ, Garner HW, et al. Clinical utility of dual-energy CT for evaluation of tophaceous gout. RadioGraphics 2011;31(5):1365–75.

39. Lormeau C, Cormier G, Sigaux J, et al. Management of septic bursitis. Joint Bone Spine 2019;86(5): 583–8.

40. Cea-Pereiro JC, Garcia-Meijide J, Mera-Varela A, et al. A comparison between septic bursitis caused by *Staphylococcus aureus* and those caused by other organisms. Clin Rheumatol 2001;20(1):10–4.

41. Baumbach SF, Lobo CM, Badyine I, et al. Prepatellar and olecranon bursitis: literature review and devel-opment of a treatment algorithm. Arch Orthop Trauma Surg 2014;134(3):359–70.

42. Hayeri MR, Ziai P, Shehata ML, et al. Soft-tissue in-fections and their imaging mimics: from cellulitis to necrotizing fasciitis. RadioGraphics 2016;36(6): 1888–910.

43. Murphey MD, Vidal JA, Fanburg-Smith JC, et al. Im-aging of synovial chondromatosis with radiologic-pathologic correlation. Radiogr Rev Publ Radiol Soc N Am Inc 2007;27(5):1465–88.

44. Walker EA, Murphey MD, Fetsch JF. Imaging char-acteristics of tenosynovial and bursal chondromato-sis. Skeletal Radiol 2011;40(3):317–25.

45. Bui-Mansfield LT, Rohini D, Bagg M. Tenosynovial chondromatosis of the ring finger. AJR Am J Roent-genol 2005;184(4):1223–4.

46. Covall DJ, Fowble CD. Synovial chondromatosis of the biceps tendon sheath. Orthop Rev 1994; 23(11):902–5.

47. Karlin C, De Smet A, Neff J, et al. The variable man-ifestations of extraarticular synovial chondromatosis. Am J Roentgenol 1981;137(4):731–5.

48. Shallop B, Abraham JA. Synovial chondromatosis of pes anserine bursa secondary to osteochondroma. Orthopedics 2014;37(8):e735–8.

49. Boya H, Pinar H, Özcan Ö. Synovial osteochondro-matosis of the suprapatellar bursa with an imperfo-rate suprapatellar plica. Arthrosc J Arthrosc Relat Surg 2002;18(4):1–3.

50. Lin Y-C, Goldsmith JD, Gebhardt MG, et al. Bursal synovial chondromatosis formation following osteo-chondroma resection. Skeletal Radiol 2014;43(7): 997–1000.

51. Stephan SR, Shallop B, Lackman R, et al. Pigmented villonodular synovitis: a comprehensive review and proposed treatment algorithm. JBJS Rev 2016;4(7).

52. Mastboom MJL, Palmerini E, Verspoor FGM, et al. Surgical outcomes of patients with diffuse-type teno-synovial giant-cell tumours: an international, retro-spective, cohort study. Lancet Oncol 2019;20(6): 877–86.

53. Murphey MD, Rhee JH, Lewis RB, et al. Pigmented villonodular synovitis: radiologic-pathologic correla-tion. Radiogr Rev Publ Radiol Soc N Am Inc 2008; 28(5):1493–518.

54. Garner HW, Ortiguera CJ, Nakhleh RE. Pigmented villonodular synovitis. RadioGraphics 2008;28(5): 1519–23.

55. Kim D-E, Kim J-M, Lee B-S, et al. Distinct extra-articular invasion patterns of diffuse pigmented villo-nodular synovitis/tenosynovial giant cell tumor in the knee joints. Knee Surg Sports Traumatol Arthrosc 2018;26(11):3508–14.

56. Sugita T, Itaya N, Aizawa T, et al. Surgical approach to pigmented villonodular synovitis and synovial os-teochondromatosis in pathological expansion of the popliteus bursa. Arthrosc Tech 2019;8(12):e1495–9.

57. Zhao H, Maheshwari AV, Kumar D, et al. Giant cell tumor of the pes anserine bursa (extra-articular pig-mented villonodular bursitis): a case report and re-view of the literature. Case Rep Med 2011;2011: 491470.

58. Maheshwari AV, Muro-Cacho CA, Pitcher JD. Pig-mented villonodular bursitis/diffuse giant cell tumor of the pes anserine bursa: a report of two cases and review of literature. The Knee 2007;14(5):402–7.

59. Coll JP, Ragsdale BD, Chow B, et al. Best cases from the AFIP: lipoma arborescens of the knees in a patient with rheumatoid arthritis. Radiogr Rev Publ Radiol Soc N Am Inc 2011;31(2):333–7.

60. Murphey MD, Carroll JF, Flemming DJ, et al. From the archives of the AFIP: benign musculoskeletal lipomatous lesions. RadioGraphics 2004;24(5): 1433–66.

61. Kalia V, Daher O, Garvin G, et al. Synchronous bilat-eral lipoma arborescens of bicipitoradial bursa: a rare entity. Skeletal Radiol 2018;47(10):1425–9.

62. Moukaddam H, Smitaman E, Haims AH. Lipoma ar-borescens of the peroneal tendon sheath. J Magn Reson Imaging JMRI 2011;33(1):221–4.

63. White EA, Omid R, Matcuk GR, et al. Lipoma arbor-escens of the biceps tendon sheath. Skeletal Radiol 2013;42(10):1461–4.

64. Kord Valeshabad A, De La Vara D, Shamim E, et al. Lipoma arborescens of the bicipitoradial bursa. Skeletal Radiol 2018;47(4):549–51.

65. Doyle AJ, Miller MV, French JG. Lipoma arborescens in the bicipital bursa of the elbow: MRI findings in two cases. Skeletal Radiol 2002;31(11):656–60.

66. Kurihashi A, Yamaguchi T, Tamai K, et al. Lipoma arborescens with osteochondral metaplasia-a case mimicking synovial osteochondromatosis in a lateral knee bursa. Acta Orthop Scand 1997;68(3):304–6.

67. Minami S, Miyake Y, Kinoshita H. Lipoma arborescens arising in the extra-articular bursa of the knee joint. SICOT-J. 2016;2:28.

68. Friedman MV, Kyriakos M, Matava MJ, et al. Intra-articular synovial sarcoma. Skeletal Radiol 2013; 42(6):859–67.

69. Murphey MD, Gibson MS, Jennings BT, et al. Imaging of synovial sarcoma with radiologic-pathologic correlation. RadioGraphics 2006;26(5):1543–65.

70. Bakri A, Shinagare AB, Krajewski KM, et al. Synovial sarcoma: imaging features of common and uncommon primary sites, metastatic patterns, and treatment response. Am J Roentgenol 2012;199(2): W208–15.

71. Dardick I, O'Brien PK, Jeans MT, et al. Synovial sarcoma arising in an anatomical bursa. Virchows Arch A Pathol Anat Histol 1982;397(1):93–101.

72. Zeiss J, Coombs RJ, Booth RL, et al. Chronic bursitis presenting as a mass in the pes anserine bursa: MR diagnosis. J Comput Assist Tomogr 1993;17(1): 137–40.

73. Di Sante L, Paoloni M, Ioppolo F, et al. Ultrasound-guided aspiration and corticosteroid injection of Baker's cysts in knee osteoarthritis: a prospective observational study. Am J Phys Med Rehabil 2010; 89(12):970–5.

74. Mortada M, Amer YA, Zaghlol RS. Efficacy and safety of musculoskeletal ultrasound guided aspiration and intra-lesional corticosteroids injection of ruptured Baker's cyst: a retrospective observational study. Clin Med Insights Arthritis Musculoskelet Disord 2020;13. 1179544120967383.

Preoperative and Postoperative Magnetic Resonance Imaging of the Cruciate Ligaments

Fangbai Wu, MD*, Ceylan Colak, MD, Naveen Subhas, MD, MPH

KEYWORDS

- Anterior cruciate ligament • Posterior cruciate ligament • MR imaging
- Anterior cruciate ligament reconstruction • Posterior cruciate ligament reconstruction

KEY POINTS

- MR imaging is highly accurate in the assessment of acute complete cruciate ligament tears but less accurate for the diagnosis of partial and chronic tears.
- Ramps lesions and anterolateral ligament injury are associated with ACL rupture and may contribute to persistent instability after ACL reconstruction
- Posterior tibial translation measured in the midmedial compartment on routine knee MR imaging may be a helpful secondary finding of chronic PCL tear and PCL graft failure.
- MR imaging is well suited for evaluation of postoperative complications following ACL and PCL reconstruction.

INTRODUCTION

The anterior cruciate ligament (ACL) and posterior cruciate ligament (PCL) are key stabilizers of the knee. Magnetic resonance (MR) imaging excels at depiction of injury in both the native and reconstructed cruciate ligaments as well as associated injuries. This article reviews the anatomy, injury patterns, and relevant surgical techniques crucial to making accurate interpretation of MR imaging of the cruciate ligaments.

NORMAL ANATOMY AND IMAGING APPEARANCE OF THE ANTERIOR CRUCIATE LIGAMENT

The ACL is an intra-articular extrasynovial structure that acts as the primary restraint to anterior tibial translation and also provides restraint to internal rotation.[1] The ACL extends from the posterior inner surface of the lateral femoral condyle to the anterior tibial plateau, anterolateral to the medial tibial spine. The ACL can be divided into 2 functional bundles named by their relative insertions on the tibia, the anteromedial bundle (AMB) and the posterolateral bundle (PLB). The bundles are roughly parallel in knee extension with the PLB providing restraint against anterior tibial translation as well as internal rotation of the tibia.[2] The bundles rotate around each other during knee flexion and the AMB becomes taut, acting to restrain anterior translation.[2]

The normal ACL demonstrates low signal intensity on T1- and T2-weighted sequences with heterogeneous striations commonly seen. In the sagittal plane, with the knee imaged in relative extension, the ACL is taut and roughly parallels the roof of the intercondylar notch (Blumensaat line) (**Fig. 1**A). The proximal ACL demonstrates an elongated ovoid shape in the axial plane at the level of the upper intercondylar notch and fans out progressively toward its tibial attachment. The femoral attachment is best seen on axial and coronal (**Fig. 1**B) sequences. The AMB and the

Department of Radiology, Imaging Institute, Cleveland Clinic, 9500 Euclid Avenue, Cleveland, OH 44195, USA
* Corresponding author.
E-mail address: wuf@ccf.org

Magn Reson Imaging Clin N Am 30 (2022) 261–275
https://doi.org/10.1016/j.mric.2021.11.006

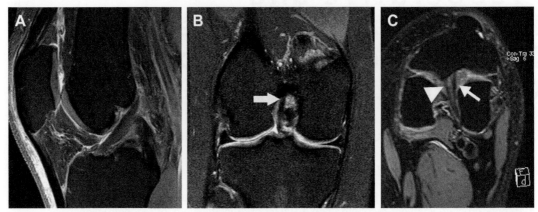

Fig. 1. Normal appearance of the ACL. Sagittal proton density (PD) fat-suppressed MR image (*A*) showing taut ACL with normal striations and heterogeneous signal intensity. Normal course of the ACL parallel to Blumensaat line is well demonstrated. Coronal PD fat-suppressed image (*B*) showing the femoral attachment of the ACL (*arrow*). Three-dimensional isotropic fast-spin echo multi-planar reformation image (*C*) in the coronal oblique plane of ACL shows delineation of the anteromedial (*arrowhead*) and posterolateral bundles (*arrow*).

PLB can be identified on axial, coronal, and oblique coronal planes (prescribed on the line of the ACL in the sagittal plane), whereas the individual bundles are often difficult to delineate and are best seen on the coronal plane near the tibial attachment (**Fig. 1**C).

Anterior Cruciate Ligament Injuries

Tears of the ACL are common with an incidence of 68.8 per 100,000 persons-years.[3] Multiple mechanisms of injury have been described, many of which involve a combination of multiplanar forces commonly seen with athletic maneuvers, including deceleration and directional movements. MR imaging is well suited for detection of ACL tears and associated injuries with sensitivity of 83% to 95% and specificity of 93% to 95% for complete ACL tears.[4] Partial tears constitute 15% of all ACL injuries.[5] MR imaging is less accurate for detection of partial tears with an accuracy rate as low as 25% to 53%.[6]

Magnetic Resonance Imaging Findings of Anterior Cruciate Ligament Injury

Acute complete tears

Although protocols vary across institutions, the typical protocol should include a combination of fluid-sensitive and T1-weighted sequences in all 3 traditional orthogonal planes. Three-dimensional (3D) isotropic fast-spin echo sequences are able to provide reformats in a multitude of oblique planes and are often helpful in challenging cases. Tears of the ACL are most commonly midsubstance but may also occur at

its femoral, or less commonly, tibial attachments.[7] **Table 1** compares the imaging features of acute complete (**Fig. 2**), partial (**Fig. 3**), and chronic tears (**Fig. 4**).

The primary MR imaging findings of acute complete ACL tear include the following:

- Focal discontinuity of fibers (see **Fig. 2**A)
- Increased intrasubstance signal on fluid-sensitive sequences
- Masslike tissue in the expected location of the ACL without normally oriented fibers
- Abnormal orientation or bowing of fibers

Discontinuity of fibers is often best depicted on axial and sagittal planes, and an empty notch sign best appreciated on coronal and axial sequences (see **Fig. 2**B). A discontinuous ACL and/or an abnormal horizontal orientation of the ACL have been shown to have 100% positive predictive value for ACL tear.[8] The most common combination of findings are diffusely increased signal and enlargement of the ACL with focal discontinuity.[8,9]

Mucoid degeneration and ganglia of the ACL are common and often coexist; they are not associated with instability[10] but may cause mechanical symptoms such as loss of full extension, and occasionally require intervention. In the case of mucoid degeneration, the ACL will be diffusely increased in signal and thickened, with normally oriented intact fibers forming regular striations (**Fig. 5**A). Ganglion cysts will be well-circumscribed fluid signal abnormalities with long axis oriented along the length of the ACL rather than transversely as seen with tears (**Fig. 5**B).

Table 1
Features of anterior cruciate ligament tears

	Acute Complete Tear	Acute Partial Tear	Chronic Tear
Fiber discontinuity/ irregularity	+	+	+/−
Increased T2 signal	+	+	-
Bone contusions	+	+/−	-
Abnormal orientation of fibers	+	+	+

Secondary findings of ACL rupture include the following:

- Osseous injuries involving the anterior aspect of the lateral femoral condyle and the posterior aspect of the lateral tibial plateau (see **Fig. 2**C)
- Less commonly, injuries may also occur in the posterior aspect of the medial tibial plateau and medial femoral condyle
- Anterior tibial translation
- Uncovering of the posterior horn of the lateral meniscus

Osseous injuries are often marrow contusions but may be associated with impaction deformities or subchondral trabecular fractures. Secondary findings are lacking in sensitivity but have high specificity for ACL rupture. Bone contusions in the lateral compartment, anterior tibial translation greater than 5 mm, and uncovering of the posterior horn of the lateral meniscus greater than 3.5 mm have specificity for ACL tear of 100%, 93%, and 100%, respectively.[11,12]

Partial tears

MR imaging is less accurate in the evaluation of partial tears compared with acute complete tears.

Distinguishing partial and complete tears and defining bundle involvement is often difficult. Partial tears may exhibit similar findings as complete tears but with the presence of definable intact fibers (see **Fig. 3**A). Other findings include attenuation, posterior bowing, and distortion of the ACL without focal discontinuity. Bone contusions are often absent (see **Fig. 3**B). Although treatment decisions take into consideration imaging, physical examination findings, and patient characteristics, partial tears involving greater than 50% of fibers are typically treated surgically at our institution.

Chronic tears

Detection of chronic tears of the ACL is often difficult. The ACL begins to heal by forming variable amount of scar tissue following the acute injury, and increased T2 signal will gradually resolve. Scar tissue is hypointense on all sequences and lacks the normal striated fibrillar pattern seen with normal ACL fibers. Scar may bridge the torn fragments and obscure the tear entirely. Laxity and abnormal horizontal orientation of fibers are the most useful features for detecting ACL disruption in the chronic setting as opposed to fiber discontinuity and bone contusions, which are the most useful features in the acute setting (see

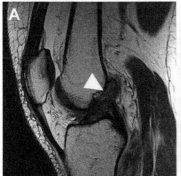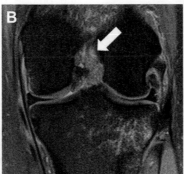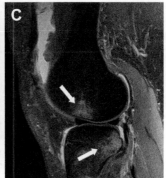

Fig. 2. Acute complete and partial tears of the ACL. Sagittal T2-weighted MR image (*A*) of the ACL with complete discontinuity of the fibers (*arrowhead*), consistent with acute complete ACL tear. Coronal proton density (PD) fat-suppressed image (*B*) showing an "empty notch" (*arrow*) with lack of intact fibers. Sagittal PD fat-suppressed image (*C*) showing kissing contusion (*arrows*).

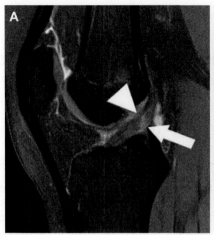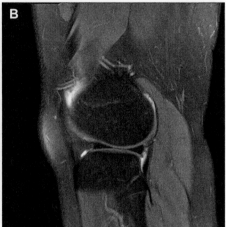

Fig. 3. High-grade partial tear of the ACL. Sagittal T2-weighted MR image (*A*) of the ACL demonstrating partial disruption of the majority of fibers (*arrow*) and a few intact fiberse anteriorly (*arrowhead*). Sagittal proton density fat-suppressed MR image (*B*) showing lack of kissing contusions.

Fig. 4). Scar most commonly attaches to the lateral aspect of the proximal PCL and the intercondylar notch, less commonly to the anatomic origin of the ACL.[13] Although the ACL may regain continuity through scar, the healed ligament will remain functionally weaker.[14] Nonvisualization of the ACL has also been described as a finding of chronic ACL tears but is relatively uncommon.[13]

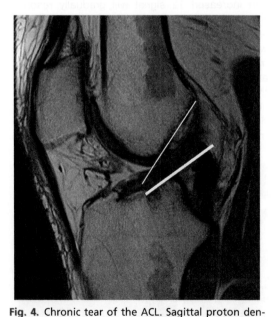

Fig. 4. Chronic tear of the ACL. Sagittal proton density MR image showing chronic tear of the ACL with attenuation of the ACL at the femoral attachment without discrete full-thickness defect. There is bowing of the fibers, which demonstrates a more horizontal course (*thick line*) relative to Blumensaat line (*thin line*).

Associated Injuries

A variety of injuries are commonly seen in conjunction with ACL tears. In addition to the aforementioned bone injuries, these include meniscus tears, injury of the medial collateral ligament (MCL), injury to the posterolateral corner structures, and avulsion of the anterolateral ligament (ALL) also termed Segond fracture. Although most of these injuries are well known and described, meniscal ramp lesions and injury of the ALL deserve further discussion in the following sections.

Ramp lesions

Vertical tears in the peripheral posterior horn of the medial meniscus or disruption of the peripheral meniscocapsular attachments occurring in conjunction with ACL tears have been termed ramp lesions, although there is disagreement on the precise definition.[15] Biomechanical studies have shown the contribution of ramp lesions to persistent instability in the ACL-deficient knee to anterior tibial translation and external rotation[16]; furthermore, these types of instabilities persisted after ACL repair alone but resolve with ACL repair plus repair of ramp lesions.[16] Although there is disagreement in surgical literature on the need to address ramp lesions in the setting of acute ACL tear, there is little dispute on the need to repair ramp lesions in the setting of chronic ACL deficiency.[17] Diagnosis is often difficult, however, as sensitivity and specificity of MR imaging have been as low as 48% and 79%, respectively, and sensitivity for arthroscopy through standard anterior portals is as low as 0% to 38%.[18] Radiologists must be aware of the imaging appearance of ramp

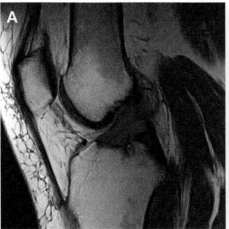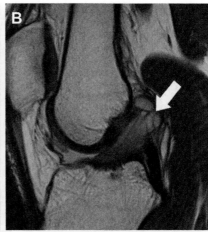

Fig. 5. Mucoid degeneration and ganglion cysts of the ACL. Sagittal proton density MR image (*A*) showing mucoid degeneration of the ACL, which is thickened and increased in signal but demonstrates normal course of intact fibers, creating a striated appearance. Sagittal T2-weighted image (*B*) showing well-defined ganglion cysts (*arrow*) along femoral attachment and coexisting mucoid degeneration.

lesions and have high suspicion in the context of concurrent ACL injury to improve preoperative diagnosis.

The following are the imaging findings of ramp lesions:

- Longitudinal vertical tear in the red-red zone of the posterior horn of the medial meniscus[19] (**Fig. 6**A, B).
- Thin fluid signal completely interposed between the posterior horn of the medial meniscus and the posteromedial capsule,[20] which has been termed meniscocapsular separation in the radiology literature (**Fig. 6**C, D).
- Irregularity at the posterior margin of the medial meniscus associated with focal contour abnormalities in the peripheral posterior horn and the meniscocapsular attachments.[21]
- Perimeniscal fluid signal intensity in the posteromedial corner.[19]
- Edema signal between the medial meniscus and medial collateral ligament.[19]

Yeo and colleagues[21] found that the most sensitive findings for ramp lesion included complete fluid filling and irregularity at the posterior margin of the medial meniscus. In the pediatric population, peripheral irregularity is a sensitive finding; however, fluidlike junctional signal was less sensitive but highly specific.[22]

Anterolateral ligament

ALL injury is frequently associated with ACL injuries. There has been much debate on the anatomic features of the ALL and its role in persistent rotational instability in the ACL-deficient knee.

Despite this, anatomic studies of the ALL have consistently identified this structure in nearly all specimens as a triangular, anterolateral structure deep to the iliotibial band.[23] The femoral origin of the ALL is located just posterior and proximal to the lateral epicondyle; its major insertion is on the proximal tibia just behind Gerdy tubercle; some fibers also insert directly onto the lateral meniscus and the anterolateral capsule.[23] The ALL is an important secondary stabilizer resisting excessive internal rotation and anterior tibial translation. For this reason, a combined ACL and ALL reconstruction may result in lower rates of graft failure as well as improved patient outcomes.[23,24]

Visibility of the ALL is variable, ranging from 51% to 100% of cases, with the distal tibial portion being the most consistently visualized[25] and often best depicted on coronal sequences (**Fig. 7**). Injuries of the ALL can occur proximally or distally, or occur in the form of a distal avulsion fracture (Segond fracture) (**Fig. 8**). The accuracy of MR imaging for identification of ALL injury in the setting of concurrent ACL injury is as high as 88%, but there is evidence that sensitivity decreases for subacute (>1 month) and chronic injuries.[26,27]

THE POSTOPERATIVE ANTERIOR CRUCIATE LIGAMENT
Surgical Management

Complete tears involving the substance of the ACL rarely heal and often require surgical intervention to reestablish stability. ACL reconstruction is the gold standard, although newer repair techniques have shown promise.[28] Double bundle reconstruction has been reported to have fewer

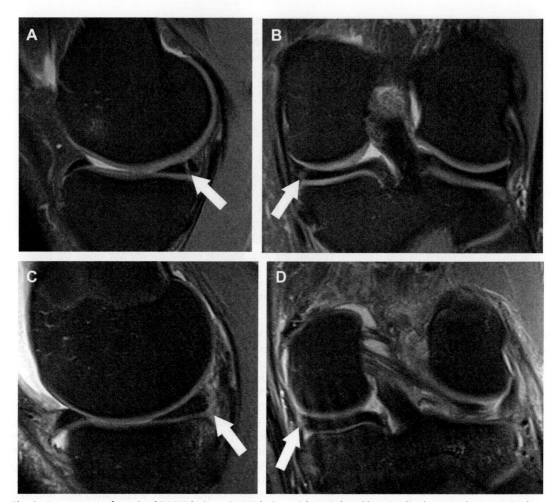

Fig. 6. Appearance of meniscal RAMP lesions. RAMP lesion with peripheral longitudinal tear in the posterior horn of the medial meniscus on the sagittal (*A*) and coronal (*B*) proton density (PD) fat-suppressed MR images (*arrows*). RAMP lesion with meniscocapsular injury; sagittal (*C*) and coronal (*D*) PD fat-suppressed images demonstrate increased signal interposed between the posterior horn of the medial meniscus and the capsule with irregularity along the posterior surface of the medial meniscus (*arrows*).

complications than single bundle reconstructions in which only the AMB is reconstructed[29]; however, single bundle reconstructions remain much more commonly performed.

Both autografts and allografts are used. Synthetic grafts are no longer commonly used because of high failure rates.[30] Allograft choices include bone-patellar-bone (BPTB) grafts as well as hamstring, posterior tibialis, and Achilles tendon grafts.

The most common choices for autografts are as follows:

- BPTB and hamstring autografts:
  ○ Harvested from the central third of the patellar tendon with bone grafts from the inferior pole of the patella and tibial tuberosity.

○ Bone grafts are initially anchored within the tunnels using interference screws but achieve deeper fixation through bone-to-bone healing, known to occur as early as 16 weeks following surgery.[28]
○ Higher rates of harvest site complications including anterior knee pain, patellar fracture, patellar tendon rupture, and arthrofibrosis.[31]

- Hamstring tendon (HT) grafts
  ○ The distal semitendinosus and gracilis tendons are common choices for HT autografts.
  ○ Grafts are anchored with a variety of surgical devices including interference screws, endobuttons, and staples. Healing of soft tissue grafts depends on progressive mineralization of fibrovascular interface

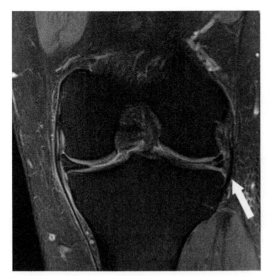

Fig. 7. Normal ALL. Coronal proton density fat-suppressed MR image showing the tibial portion of the ALL (*arrow*), the most consistently visualized part of the ALL.

and subsequent bone incorporation into the outer tendon, which eventually results in a fibrous insertion of the tendon, a process that may take up to 12 months.[28]

○ HT grafts may have less donor site complications compared with BPTB grafts but higher rates of weakness in full extension,

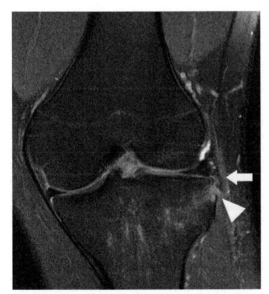

Fig. 8. Injury of the ALL with associated Segond fracture. Coronal proton density fat-suppressed MR image showing injury of the ALL, which demonstrates increased signal (*arrow*) and a small associated avulsion fracture (*arrowhead*) of the tibia.

terminal knee flexion, graft laxity, and higher infection rate.[31]

○ Harvested HT regeneration is common, as high as up to 86% of the time.[32]

● Quadriceps tendon autografts are gaining in popularity due to lower harvest site morbidity than BPTB grafts and better functional outcomes than hamstring grafts with comparable graft survival rate.[31]

Regardless of the graft choice, optimal tunnel placement is vital for normal function of the graft. The tibial tunnel should be placed such that the graft parallels Blumensaat line with the knee in extension. A too-vertical orientation of the graft may predispose to PCL impingement and rotational instability.[33] Physeal-sparing, partial transphyseal, and transphyseal methods of reconstructions have been used in the skeletally immature population. Physeal-sparing techniques are favored in the younger population with a large amount of growth remaining.[34] For transphyseal methods, vertical tunnels may minimize the area of the physis traversed but must be weighed against a less anatomic reconstruction.[34]

Normal Postoperative Appearance of the Anterior Cruciate Ligament

The ACL graft heals by undergoing a period of necrosis followed by revascularization, remodeling, and finally, ligamentization. The graft will demonstrate intermediate to high signal during the earlier phases, eventually becoming homogeneously dark after complete ligamentization, which takes 12 to 24 months (**Fig. 9**).

Normal postoperative appearance of ACL reconstruction:

● Uniform caliber and regular arrangement of graft fibers with course parallel to Blumensaat line.

● Intermediate to high T1 and T2 signal of the graft before ligamentization, which typically occurs by 18 months. Fairly uniform T1 and T2 signal similar to the native ACL will be seen in a ligamentized graft.

● Trace amount of fluid may be seen between strands of HT grafts.

● Central defect in the patellar tendon with BPTB harvest, which typically fills with scar by 2 years postoperatively; thereafter there is often persistent thinning in the harvest site with thickened appearance of the surrounding patellar tendon.[35]

● Partial or even complete-appearing regeneration of harvested HTs may be seen.

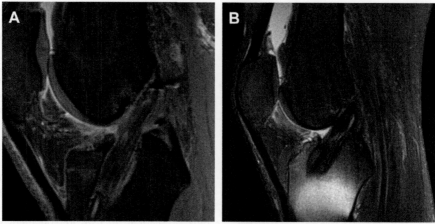

Fig. 9. Normal appearance of the postoperative ACL. Sagittal proton density fat-suppressed MR images showing intermediate signal of nonligamentized graft less than 2 years postoperatively (*A*) and low homogeneous signal intensity of the ligamentized graft 3 years after surgery (*B*).

Complications of Anterior Cruciate Ligament Reconstruction

Aside from donor site complications touched upon earlier and postsurgical infection, several other complications can occur following ACL reconstruction surgery.

Graft tear

Patients with graft tear present with recurrent instability, often with accompanying history of recent injury. MR imaging is 87.5% accurate for diagnosis of complete graft tears and 37.5% accurate for diagnosis of partial tears.[36] Perhaps the greatest value of MR imaging is in the exclusion of graft tears. Absence of graft discontinuity or caliber change has 100% negative predictive value for graft tear.[36]

The following are the MR imaging findings of graft tear:

- Complete or partial graft discontinuity (**Figs. 10** and **11**)
- Focal change in the caliber of the graft
- Posterior bowing of the graft, although this may also be seen with graft stretching and laxity
- Secondary signs similar to native ACL tears such as "kissing contusions"

Table 2 compares the normal and abnormal appearance of the ACL graft.

Graft impingement

Patients with graft impingement may present with loss of range of motion, most commonly full extension, and may be predisposed to graft tearing. Roof impingement is a term used most often to describe ACL graft impingement caused by a tibial tunnel placed too anteriorly (partially or completely anterior to the intersection of Blumensaat line) but may also be seen as a result of abnormal mechanics secondary to the presence of a notch osteophyte (**Fig. 12**A). MR findings will include contact between the anterior aspect of the ACL graft with the roof of the intercondylar notch with possible posterior deformation of the graft by the anterior inferior edge of the intercondylar roof. Increased signal intensity may be seen within the distal two-thirds of the graft.[37]

Arthrofibrosis

Patients with arthrofibrosis following ACL reconstruction may present with stiffness or restricted extension similar to that of graft impingement. Scar may develop focally, forming the so-called cyclops lesion, which appears as a fibrotic nodular mass in the anterior intercondylar notch (**Fig. 12**B). Arthrofibrosis may also surround the graft or appear as low-signal scarring within Hoffa fat pad. Occasionally, partially torn graft fibers are displaced into the intercondylar notch, creating an appearance similar to a cyclops lesion, which has been termed "pseudo-cyclops lesion."[38] As opposed to a true cyclops lesion, a portion of the involved fibers can be seen extending into the tibial or femoral tunnels.

Ganglion cyst formation and tunnel widening

Ganglion cysts may form either within the graft or the tibial tunnel. Although ganglion cysts are not associated with graft failure, cysts may be symptomatic from mass effect, requiring debridement or aspiration. Ganglion cysts may be more commonly seen with HT grafts and endobutton

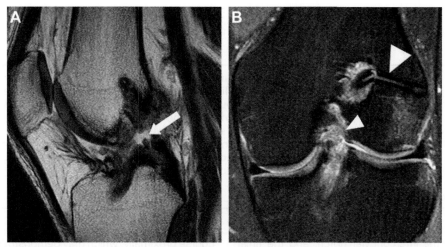

Fig. 10. Complete tear of the ACL graft and fractured hardware. Sagittal T2-weighted MR image (*A*) demonstrating complete graft tear with a gap (*arrow*) between fibers. Coronal proton density fat-suppressed image (*B*) shows amorphous tissue at the location of ACL (*small arrowhead*) without intact fibers and broken pin (*large arrowhead*).

fixation devices.[39] Tunnel widening, however, may occur with or without ganglion cyst formation. Causes of tunnel widening include attritional bone loss related to repetitive motion of the graft within the tunnel and granulomatous reactions related to bioabsorbable anchors, which have fallen out of favor for this reason. Tibial tunnel between 10 and 16 mm diameter is abnormal and may need grafting. A tibial tunnel greater than 16 mm in diameter will always need grafting.[39]

Hardware failure
Hardware failure may include hardware fracture (see **Fig. 10**B), dislodgement, and malpositioning. Fractured and dislodged hardware may lead to

mechanical symptoms. Failure of graft fixation may occur if hardware fails before incorporation of the graft. Malpositioned hardware or displaced broken hardware fragments may cause mechanical impingement or irritation of surrounding structures.

NORMAL ANATOMY AND IMAGING APPEARANCE OF THE POSTERIOR CRUCIATE LIGAMENT

The PCL functions as the primary restraint to posterior tibial translation and aids in resisting internal rotation with knee flexion beyond 90°. The femoral attachment of the PCL is at the anteromedial

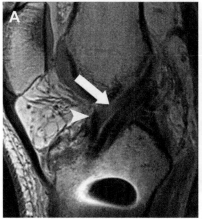
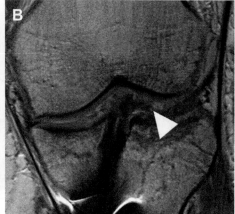

Fig. 11. Partial tear of ACL graft. Sagittal proton density (PD) MR image (*A*) showing partial disruption of the fibers (*arrow*) with anterolaterally flipped torn fibers (*arrowhead*). Coronal PD image (*B*) again showing anterolaterally displaced torn fibers (*arrowhead*).

Table 2
Post-operative appearance and complications of the anterior cruciate ligament reconstruction

Normal	Tear	Other Complications
• Uniform caliber and regular arrangement of fibers • Course parallel to Blumensaat line • Ligamentization and uniform Tl- and T2-hypointense signal of the graft by 24 mo • Variable intermediate signal of the graft before full ligamentization	• Discontinuous graft or focal change in caliber of graft • Abnormal course of fibers • Irregularity of fibers and increased T2 signal in previously ligamentized graft • Bone contusions accompany high-grade acute graft tears	• Graft impingement related to suboptimal tunnel placement or notch osteophyte • Arthrofibrosis/cyclops lesion • Hardware failure • Ganglion cyst formation and tunnel widening

aspect of the intercondylar notch, and the tibial attachment is at the midline of the tibial plateau, just below the joint line. It is made up of 2 functional bundles named based on their relative femoral attachments, the larger anterolateral bundle (ALB) and a smaller posteromedial bundle (PMB). The bundles have a codominant role in resisting posterior tibial translation at all angles of flexion, although the ALB is more active at 70° to 105° of flexion and the PMB is more active between 0° and 15° and deep extension.[40,41] The PCL is functionally supported by the anterior (Humphrey) and posterior (Wrisberg) meniscofemoral ligaments as well as the posterolateral corner structures.[40]

On MR imaging, the normal PCL demonstrates homogeneously low signal intensity on all pulse sequences (**Fig. 13**A). The PCL has a more vertical course distally and a more curved horizontal course proximally, which may demonstrate slightly increased signal on T1-weighted sequences due to magic angle artifact; this will not have corresponding signal abnormality on longer echo time sequences. The PCL is well visualized throughout its course on sagittal sequences. The axial and coronal sequences allow further assessment of the proximal and distal segments, respectively, relating to the morphology of the PCL.

POSTERIOR CRUCIATE LIGAMENT INJURIES

Injury of the PCL occurs in 38% of acute knee injuries, with a higher incidence of 56.5% in patients with trauma and in conjunction with other ligament injuries 95% of the time.[42] Mechanisms of injury include posterior tibial force with the knee in flexion as occurs with the so-called dashboard injury in motor vehicle accidents and fall on a

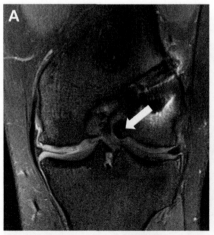
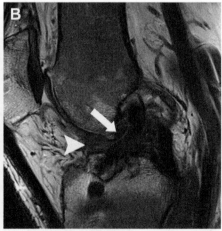

Fig. 12. Notch osteophyte causing impingement of the ACL graft and cyclops lesion. Coronal proton density fat-suppressed MR image (*A*) demonstrating notch osteophyte (*arrow*) in the intercondylar notch, protruding against the ACL graft. Sagittal T2-weighted image (*B*) demonstrating a masslike low-signal arthrofibrosis (*arrowhead*) in the anterior intercondylar notch and again notch osteophyte protruding against the ACL graft, which is posteriorly bowed.

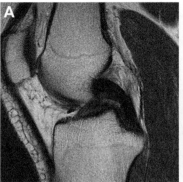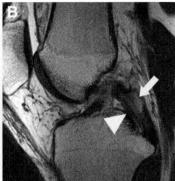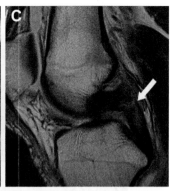

Fig. 13. Intact PCL and tears of the PCL. Sagittal intermediate weighted MR image (*A*) showing normal course and homogeneously low signal of the normal PCL. Sagittal T2-weighted image (*B*) showing partial discontinuity of posterior midfibers (*arrow*) of the PCL with intact fibers more anteriorly (*arrowhead*), consistent with partial PCL tear. Sagittal proton density image (*C*) demonstrating complete focal defect (*arrow*) in the midfibers, consistent with complete PCL tear.

hyperflexed knee. PCL injury may also occur in the setting of multiligamentous injury with severe hyperextension and/or excessive rotation. MR imaging is highly accurate for detection of acute PCL tears with sensitivity and specificity of 96% and 100% but less accurate for chronic injuries with sensitivity of 62.5%.[43]

Magnetic Resonance Imaging Findings of Posterior Cruciate Ligament Injury

Tears of the PCL are mostly midsubstance but may also occur at its femoral or tibial attachments. Bony avulsion at its tibial insertion occurs in 10% of cases.[40] Complete tears of the PCL from its femoral attachment without an associated bony avulsion have been termed "peel-off" tears and

may be repaired arthroscopically.[44] Partial tears occur more frequently in the PCL compared with the ACL. It is important to note that an acutely torn PCL will often appear as one continuous structure, in up to 62% to 75% of cases,[45,46] and differentiating between complete and partial tears is difficult. Mucoid degeneration may be confused for PCL injury, but normal course of fibers together with the presence of low-signal-intensity margins are helpful distinguishing features.

MR imaging findings of acute injury are as follows:

- Focal discontinuity of fibers (**Fig. 13**B, C)
- Greater than 7 mm anteroposterior diameter of the ligament distal to the genu on sagittal T2-weighted sequence[45]

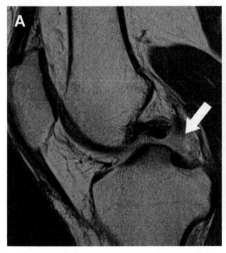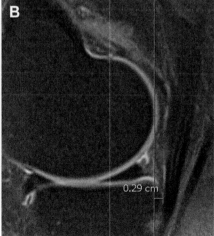

Fig. 14. Chronic tear of the PCL. Sagittal intermediate weighted image (*A*) with complete absence of the fibers (*arrow*) and posterior tibial translation, measured on sagittal proton density fat-suppressed image (*B*) in the midmedial compartment (>2 mm), a finding that is seen with tear/PCL insufficiency.

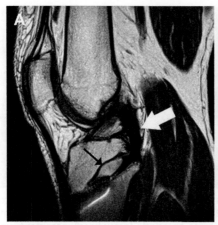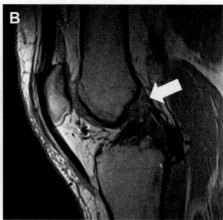

Fig. 15. Postoperative appearance of intact and torn PCL grafts. Intermediate weighted image (*A*) showing homogeneously hypointense signal of intact PCL graft (*white arrow*) and small ganglion in the tibial tunnel (*black arrow*). High-grade tear of PCL graft (*B*), marked attenuation of the PCL graft (*arrow*) distal to the femoral tunnel with increased signal and surrounding scar.

- Abnormal intermediate or fluid intrasubstance signal, which may be more pronounced on proton density images[45]
- Striated appearance of the PCL
- Lax or wavy appearance of fibers

MR imaging is limited in the detection of chronically injured and functionally deficient PCL. The chronically injured PCL can be thickened or elongated with persistently abnormal contour. Discontinuity is uncommon (**Fig. 14**A). One study found that signal abnormality following an acute injury may return to normal within 6 months; 28% of cases showed an essentially normal contour, and 44% of cases showed continuous appearance of the PCL with persistent contour abnormality.[47] Posterior tibial translation is an important finding that may point to persistent PCL deficiency and instability. Posterior tibial translation measured on sagittal sequence in the midmedial compartment of 2 to 2.9 mm on routine knee MR imaging may indicate the presence of chronic PCL injury[43,48] (**Fig. 14**B).

THE POSTOPERATIVE POSTERIOR CRUCIATE LIGAMENT
Surgical Management and Normal Postoperative Appearance

Partial isolated PCL tears are generally treated nonoperatively. Although historically isolated complete PCL tears were often not treated surgically, there is now evidence to suggest that nonoperative treatment may increase the risk of medial and patellofemoral compartment degenerative changes.[49,50] Surgical treatment is recommended for symptomatic isolated PCL tears and combined

PCL and additional ligamentous injury.[41] In cases in which a bony avulsion is present, the bone is fixed. Single bundle reconstruction of the larger ALB is traditionally performed; however, some studies have shown superior restoration of kinematic function and functional outcomes with double bundle fixation.[51,52]

Various types of grafts and surgical fixation techniques are used. The femoral tunnel is placed along the anterior aspect of the native PCL foot print in the anterior intercondylar notch.[53] Tibial tunnel placement varies between single and double bundle techniques, but care should be taken not to place it too anterior because this would risk injury to the anterior medial meniscal root.[41,54] A tibial inlay technique is typically used with BPTB graft, which involves making a trough at the tibial attachment to match the bone plug; this avoids the sharp angle the graft would have to make at the aperture of the tibial tunnel, which may damage the graft over time.

Normal Postoperative Appearance of the Posterior Cruciate Ligament

The PCL graft may have a straight or curved contour and undergoes ligamentization like ACL grafts, which is complete at 12 to 24 months[54] (**Fig. 15**A). Linear intermediate or high T2 signal may be observed between bundles of an HT graft, which usually resolves 1 to 2 years after surgery.[54]

Postoperative Complications of Posterior Cruciate Ligament Reconstruction

Complications of PCL reconstruction are similar to complications of ACL reconstruction including graft tear and stretching (**Fig. 15**B), impingement, arthrofibrosis, ganglion formation, and tunnel widening. Donor site complications and failure of fixation may also occur. Graft tears may occur through new injury or chronic impingement usually related to suboptimal tunnel positioning. MR imaging findings of graft tear are similar to that of ACL, although sensitivity has been reported to be as low as 18%.[43] Posterior tibial translation of 3.6 mm or greater measured in the midmedial compartment may be a secondary sign of graft failure.[43] The configuration of hardware, especially with the inlay technique and multiligament reconstruction, may further limit assessment of the PCL graft.

SUMMARY

MR imaging is the modality of choice for the assessment of cruciate ligament injury and postoperative complications. Radiologists should have a solid understanding of the relevant anatomy, injury patterns, surgical technique, and expected postsurgical appearance, as well as the spectrum of postoperative complications.

CLINICS CARE POINTS

- MR imaging is highly accurate and the diagnostic test of choice for detecting acute cruciate ligament injury, associated findings such as meniscus tears, and postoperative complications.
- MR imaging is less accurate for the diagnosis of partial and chronic cruciate injury, and findings in these cases should be interpreted in the context of the full clinical picture including physical examination findings.

DISCLOSURE

The authors have nothing to disclose regarding this article.

REFERENCES

1. Matsumoto H, Suda Y, Otani T, et al. Roles of the anterior cruciate ligament and the medial collateral ligament in preventing valgus instability. J Orthop Sci 2001;6(1):28–32.
2. Steckel H, Starman JS, Baums MH, et al. Anatomy of the anterior cruciate ligament double bundle structure: A macroscopic evaluation. Scand J Med Sci Sports 2007;17(4):387–92.
3. Sanders TL, Maradit Kremers H, Bryan AJ, et al. Incidence of anterior cruciate ligament tears and reconstruction: A 21-year population-based study. Am J Sports Med 2016;44(6):1502–7.
4. Phelan N, Rowland P, Galvin R, et al. A systematic review and meta-analysis of the diagnostic accuracy of MRI for suspected ACL and meniscal tears of the knee. Knee Surg Sports Traumatol Arthrosc 2016; 24(5):1525–39.
5. Buckley SL, Barrack RL, Alexander AH. The natural history of conservatively treated partial anterior cruciate ligament tears. Am J Sports Med 1989;17(2): 221–5.
6. van Dyck P, de Smet E, Veryser J, et al. Partial tear of the anterior cruciate ligament of the knee: injury patterns on MR imaging. Knee Surg Sports Traumatol Arthrosc 2012;20(2):256–61.
7. Remer EM, Fitzgerald SW, Friedman H, et al. Anterior cruciate ligament injury: MR imaging diagnosis and patterns of Injury1. Radiographics 1992;12(5): 901–15.
8. Barry KP, Mesgarzadeh M, Triolo J, et al. Accuracy of MRI patterns in evaluating anterior cruciate ligament tears. Skeletal Radiol 1996;25(4):365–70.
9. Robertson PL, Schweitzer ME, Bartolozzi AR, et al. Anterior cruciate ligament tears: evaluation of multiple signs with MR imaging. Radiology 1994;193(3): 829–34.
10. Bergin D, Morrison WB, Carrino JA, et al. Anterior cruciate ligament ganglia and mucoid degeneration: coexistence and clinical correlation. AJR Am J Roentgenol 2004;182(5):1283–7. Available at. www.ajronline.org.
11. Vahey TN, Hunt JE, Shelbourne KD. Anterior translocation of the tibia at MR imaging: a secondary sign of anterior cruciate ligament tear. Radiology 1993; 187(3):817–9.
12. Gentili A, Seeger LL, Yao L, et al. Anterior cruciate ligament tear: indirect signs at MR imaging. Radiology 1994;193(3):835–40.
13. Vahey TN, Broome DR, Kayes KJ, et al. Acute and chronic tears of the anterior cruciate ligament: Differential features at MR imaging. Radiology 1991; 181(1):251–3.
14. Frank CB. Normal ligament structure and physiology. J Musculoskelet Neuronal Interact 2004;4(2): 199–201.
15. Balazs GC, Greditzer HG, Wang D, et al. Ramp lesions of the medial meniscus in patients undergoing primary and revision ACL reconstruction: prevalence and risk factors. Orthop J Sports Med 2019; 7(5). https://doi.org/10.1177/2325967119843509.
16. Stephen JM, Halewood C, Kittl C, et al. Posteromedial meniscocapsular lesions increase tibiofemoral joint laxity with anterior cruciate ligament deficiency,

and their repair reduces laxity. Am J Sports Med 2016;44(2):400–8.

17. Chahla J, Dean CS, Moatshe G, et al. Meniscal ramp lesions: anatomy, incidence, diagnosis, and treatment. Orthop J Sports Med 2016;4(7). https://doi.org/10.1177/2325967116657815.

18. Bumberger A, Koller U, Hofbauer M, et al. Ramp lesions are frequently missed in ACL-deficient knees and should be repaired in case of instability. Knee Surg Sports Traumatol Arthrosc 2020;28(3):840–54.

19. Greif DN, Baraga MG, Rizzo MG, et al. MRI appearance of the different meniscal ramp lesion types, with clinical and arthroscopic correlation. Skeletal Radiol 2020;49(5):677–89.

20. Hash TW. Magnetic resonance imaging of the knee. Sports Health 2013;5(1):78–107.

21. Yeo Y, Ahn JM, Kim H, et al. MR evaluation of the meniscal ramp lesion in patients with anterior cruciate ligament tear. Skeletal Radiol 2018;47(12):1683–9.

22. Nguyen JC, Bram JT, Lawrence JTR, et al. MRI criteria for meniscal ramp lesions of the knee in children with anterior cruciate ligament tears. AJR Am J Roentgenol 2021;216(3):791–8.

23. Sonnery-Cottet B, Daggett M, Fayard JM, et al. Anterolateral Ligament Expert Group consensus paper on the management of internal rotation and instability of the anterior cruciate ligament - deficient knee. J Orthop Traumatol 2017;18(2):91–106.

24. Saithna A, Daggett M, Helito CP, et al. Clinical results of combined ACL and anterolateral ligament reconstruction: a narrative review from the SANTI Study Group. J Knee Surg 2020;5. https://doi.org/10.1055/s-0040-1701220.

25. Patel RM, Brophy RH. Anterolateral ligament of the knee: anatomy, function, imaging, and treatment. Am J Sports Med 2018;46(1):217–23.

26. Monaco E, Helito CP, Redler A, et al. Correlation between magnetic resonance imaging and surgical exploration of the anterolateral structures of the acute anterior cruciate ligament–injured knee. Am J Sports Med 2019;47(5):1186–93.

27. Han AX, Tan TJ, Nguyen T, et al. Timing of magnetic resonance imaging affects the accuracy and interobserver agreement of anterolateral ligament tears detection in anterior cruciate ligament deficient knees. Knee Surg Relat Res 2020;32(1):64.

28. Van Dyck P, Lambrecht V, De Smet E, et al. Imaging of the postoperative anterior cruciate ligament: emphasis on new surgical and imaging methods. In: Seminars in musculoskeletal radiology, vol. 20. Thieme Medical Publishers, Inc.; 2016. p. 33–42. https://doi.org/10.1055/s-0036-1579678.

29. Järvelä S, Kiekara T, Suomalainen P, et al. Double-bundle versus single-bundle anterior cruciate ligament reconstruction: a Prospective Randomized Study with 10-Year Results. Am J Sports Med 2017;45(11):2578–85.

30. Satora W, Królikowska A, Czamara A, et al. Synthetic grafts in the treatment of ruptured anterior cruciate ligament of the knee joint. Polim Med 2017;47(1):55–9.

31. Mouarbes D, Menetrey J, Marot V, et al. Anterior cruciate ligament reconstruction: a systematic review and meta-analysis of outcomes for quadriceps tendon autograft versus bone-patellar tendon-bone and hamstring-tendon autografts. Am J Sports Med 2019;47(14):3531–40.

32. Papalia R, Franceschi F, D'Adamio S, et al. Hamstring tendon regeneration after harvest for anterior cruciate ligament reconstruction: a systematic review. Arthroscopy 2015;31(6):1169–83.

33. Simmons R, Howell SM, Hull ML. Effect of the angle of the femoral and tibial tunnels in the coronal plane and incremental excision of the posterior cruciate ligament on tension of an anterior cruciate ligament graft: an in vitro study. J Bone Joint Surg Am 2003;85(6):1018–29.

34. Perkins CA, Willimon SC. Pediatric Anterior Cruciate Ligament Reconstruction. Orthop Clin North Am 2020;51(1):55–63.

35. Svensson M, Kartus J, Ejerhed L, et al. Does the patellar tendon normalize after harvesting its central third?: a prospective long-term MRI study. Am J Sports Med 2004;32(1):34–8.

36. Horton LK, Jacobson JA, Lin J, et al. MR imaging of anterior cruciate ligament reconstruction graft. Am J Roentgenology 2000;175(4):1091–7.

37. Howell SM, Berns GS, Farley TE. Unimpinged and impinged anterior cruciate ligament grafts: MR signal intensity measurements. Radiology 1991;179(3):639–43.

38. Simpfendorfer C, Miniaci A, Subhas N, et al. Pseudocyclops: two cases of ACL graft partial tears mimicking cyclops lesions on MRI. Skeletal Radiol 2015;44(8):1169–73.

39. Groves C, Chandramohan M, Chew C, et al. Use of CT in the management of anterior cruciate ligament revision surgery. Clin Radiol 2013;68(10):e552–9.

40. Parkar AP, Alcalá-Galiano A. Rupture of the Posterior Cruciate Ligament: Preoperative and Postoperative Assessment. In: Seminars in Musculoskeletal Radiology, vol. 20. Thieme Medical Publishers, Inc.; 2016. p. 43–51. https://doi.org/10.1055/s-0036-1579711.

41. Pache S, Aman ZS, Kennedy M, et al. Current concepts review posterior cruciate ligament: current concepts review. Arch Bone Jt Surg 2018;6(1):8–18. Available at: http://abjs.mums.ac.irtheonlineversionofthisarticleabjs.mums.ac.ir. Accessed July 11, 2021.

42. Fanelli GC, Edson CJ. Posterior cruciate ligament injuries in trauma patients: Part II. Arthroscopy 1995;11(5):526–9.

43. DePhillipo NN, Cinque ME, Godin JA, et al. Posterior tibial translation measurements on magnetic

resonance imaging improve diagnostic sensitivity for chronic posterior cruciate ligament injuries and graft tears. Am J Sports Med 2018;46(2):341–7.

44. Ross G, Driscoll J, McDevitt E, et al. Arthroscopic posterior cruciate ligament repair for acute femoral "peel off" tears. Arthroscopy 2003;19(4):431–5.

45. Rodriguez W Jr, Vinson EN, Helms CA, et al. MRI appearance of posterior cruciate ligament tears. AJR Am J Roentgenol 2008;191(4):1031.

46. Akisue T, Kurosaka M, Yoshiya S, et al. Evaluation of healing of the injured posterior cruciate ligament: Analysis of instability and magnetic resonance imaging. Arthroscopy 2001;17(3):264–9.

47. Jung YB, Jung HJ, Yang JJ. Characterization of spontaneous healing of chronic posterior cruciate ligament injury: analysis of instability and magnetic resonance imaging. J Magn Reson Imaging 2008; 27(6):1336–40.

48. Degnan AJ, Maldjian C, Adam RJ, et al. Passive posterior tibial subluxation on routine knee MRI as a secondary sign of PCL tear. Radiol Res Pract 2014;2014:1–6.

49. Boynton MD, Tietjens BR. Long-term followup of the untreated isolated posterior cruciate ligament-deficient knee. Am J Sports Med 1996;24(3): 306–10.

50. Strobel MJ, Weiler A, Schulz MS, et al. Arthroscopic evaluation of articular cartilage lesions in posterior-cruciate-ligament-deficient knees. Arthroscopy 2003;19(3):262–8.

51. Wijdicks CA, Kennedy NI, Goldsmith MT, et al. Kinematic analysis of the posterior cruciate ligament, part 2: a comparison of anatomic single- versus double-bundle reconstruction. Am J Sports Med 2013;41(12):2839–48.

52. Bergfeld JA, McAllister DR, Parker RD, et al. A biomechanical comparison of posterior cruciate ligament reconstruction techniques. Am J Sports Med 2001;29(2):129–36.

53. Christel P. Basic principles for surgical reconstruction of the PCL in chronic posterior knee instability. Knee Surg Sports Traumatol Arthrosc 2003;11(5): 289–96.

54. Alcalá-Galiano A, Baeva M, Ismael M, et al. Imaging of posterior cruciate ligament (PCL) reconstruction: normal postsurgical appearance and complications. Skeletal Radiol 2014;43(12):1659–68.

MR Imaging Knee Synovitis and Synovial Pathology

Carissa M. White, MD*, William W. Kesler, MD, Lane Miner, DO, Donald Flemming, MD

KEYWORDS

- Knee • Synovitis • Osteoarthritis

KEY POINTS

- Knee synovitis is a nonspecific finding seen in the setting of joint damage and inflammation.
- Findings of synovial thickening, joint effusion, and synovial enhancement are present across the spectrum of etiologies and do not allow a specific diagnosis in most cases.
- The most specific signs of acute infectious arthritis are diffuse bone marrow edema, adjacent soft tissue abscess, sinus tract, and osteomyelitis.
- IV contrast is helpful to distinguish joint fluid from synovial proliferation and imaging should be performed in the first few minutes after injection.

INTRODUCTION

MR imaging of the knee is the most common examination in the nonaxial skeleton performed with this modality, and synovitis is a common finding in patients presenting with knee pain. This article reviews MR imaging of the normal synovium and synovitis.

NORMAL SYNOVIAL ANATOMY AND PHYSIOLOGY

Understanding of the normal anatomy and function of the synovium provides insight into expected imaging findings. The synovium is a thin structure that lines the nonarticulating surfaces of the joint. It is a highly specialized tissue that has evolved to be deformable, porous, and nonadherent to function in a mobile joint.[1] Its main purpose is to provide nutrition to and lubrication of the articular cartilage. The synovium is comprised of two functional components: the synovial intima and the subintimal stroma.

The layer in direct communication with joint fluid is the synovial intima and is one to three cell layers thick (60 μm).[1] The dominant cells in the intima are fibroblast like synoviocytes (FLS) that are interspersed by macrophages.[2] These FLS cells are highly specialized and play a significant role in joint homeostasis through production of lubricin and matrix metalloproteinases. The subintimal stroma lies between the intima and joint capsule and is loose tissue comprised of extracellular matrix, blood vessels, fibroblasts, macrophages, and adipocytes. The distribution of specific cells and other elements of the synovium in these layers is heterogeneous in each joint. As an example, vascularity is increased at the junction of normal cartilage, ligament/capsule, and synovium.

The production and composition of synovial fluid is important for normal joint homeostasis and is regulated by the synovium and synovial vasculature. Synovial fluid volume is approximately 2.5 mL in the normal knee.[2] It is mainly a combination of protein-rich plasma ultrafiltrate and hyaluronan and lubricin produced by FLS cells. It contains glucose that is actively transported across the synovium and thus provides nutrition to cartilage. Clearance of joint fluid is accomplished by lymphatics, which is aided by joint motion.

The dynamic nature of the knee joint leads to wear and tear of normal tissue, which necessitates mechanisms for repair and remodeling of articular cartilage and bone and mechanisms to shut down these processes to maintain joint health.

Penn State Health Milton S. Hershey Medical Center, 500 University Drive, MCH066, Hershey, PA 17033, USA
* Corresponding author.
E-mail address: cwhite8@pennstatehealth.psu.edu

Magn Reson Imaging Clin N Am 30 (2022) 277–291
https://doi.org/10.1016/j.mric.2021.11.007

Homeostasis of the joint is regulated by cytokines, growth factors, and matrix metalloproteinases.

ABNORMAL SYNOVIAL PHYSIOLOGY

The synovium has two possible temporal responses at a macroscopic level to joint injury depending on the cause.[3] The acute response may be limited to increased blood flow in preexisting vessels, and the subacute to chronic response includes synovial proliferation with vascular proliferation. Synovial blood flow is regulated by intrinsic and extrinsic factors that include neural and humoral influences. Hyperemia leads to changes in the extracellular matrix and joint effusion. Joint effusion is a sensitive but nonspecific finding of joint pathology because its formation is not reliant on the presence of synovitis. Depending on the inciting event, increased blood flow may be followed by, or coincide with, the development of synovitis. Synovitis manifests macroscopically as hyperplasia and hyperemia. Histologically it has varying degrees of three findings depending on the cause of the synovitis: (1) hyperplasia of intima, (2) increase in number and type of cells and angiogenesis in the subintimal stroma, and (3) inflammatory cell infiltration.[4] Although the cause of synovitis may be histologically definable in some cases, macroscopically it is usually indistinguishable.

NORMAL MAGNETIC RESONANCE IMAGING APPEARANCE OF SYNOVIUM

Normal synovium is indistinguishable from joint fluid on fat-saturated T2-weighted and STIR images, becoming evident only after intravenous (IV) contrast administration. It is less than 2 mm thick and demonstrates smooth and uniform contrast enhancement.[5] Synovium envelops the cruciate ligaments, which are extrasynovial structures, and extends along the popliteus tendon sheath, and so thin enhancement along these structures should not be interpreted as abnormal (**Fig. 1**). Synovium also extends into a Baker cyst if present. Normal knee synovium has intra-articular folds, or plica, which traverse the suprapatellar and medial knee joint, and across the infrapatellar (Hoffa) fat pad. Synovium lining plica enhance the same as normal synovium lining the joint capsule.

MAGNETIC RESONANCE IMAGING PROTOCOLS FOR IMAGING OF SYNOVIUM

Protocol for imaging of synovitis is predicated on the indication for imaging. Routine knee MR imaging is usually performed as a noncontrast examination for the indication of pain, with a sagittal proton density weighted sequence and fluid-sensitive sequences in sagittal, coronal, and axial planes. Synovitis can sometimes be appreciated on standard fluid-sensitive sequences, such as T2 fast spin echo without fat saturation, intermediate fast spin echo with fat saturation, and T2 fast spin echo with fat saturation. However, an additional postcontrast fat-saturated T1-weighted sequence in one or two planes (axial or sagittal) is necessary to document the extent of acute synovitis. IV contrast is particularly recommended in the evaluation of suspected rheumatoid arthritis (RA),[6,7] seronegative spondyloarthropathy (SpA),[7] and infection.[8] The postcontrast sequence should be acquired less than 5 minutes after contrast administration.[6] Dynamic contrast-enhanced MR imaging shows promise in investigational studies for the evaluation of synovitis in knee osteoarthritis (KOA), showing better correlation with pain scores than conventional static MR imaging.[6] However, at this time, dynamic contrast-enhanced MR imaging remains investigational and not practical for use in routine clinical imaging.

ABNORMAL SYNOVIUM ON MAGNETIC RESONANCE IMAGING

Synovitis is often, but not always, accompanied by a joint effusion. Most authors agree that synovial thickening cannot be reliably distinguished from joint fluid on unenhanced MR imaging[9–11]; however, because it can be variably recognized, and because most routine knee MR imaging is noncontrast, the practicing radiologist needs to be able to assess synovitis either way. Singson and Zalduondo[12] reported that in two-thirds of their cases, synovial thickening was mildly hypointense to joint fluid on fat-saturated T2-weighted and STIR images, which is theorized to be caused by fibrosis or prior intrasynovial hemorrhage in chronic synovitis.[13] They found that synovitis was isointense to joint fluid on fluid-sensitive images about one-third of the time,[12] becoming evident only after IV contrast administration. In these cases, the hyperintensity of the thickened synovium is thought to result from the increased water content seen in acute inflammation.[13,14] In chronic synovitis, there may be little joint fluid present, which is evident on postcontrast images when nearly the entirely of the intra-articular T2 bright signal is shown to enhance (**Fig. 2**). Thickened synovium is intermediate in signal on T1-weighted non-fat-suppressed images, and is distinguished from more hypointense joint fluid[12]; however, this sequence is not usually included in routine knee MR imaging.

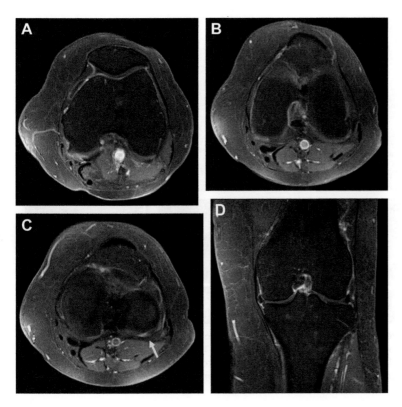

Fig. 1. Normal synovium. Post-contrast axial (*A–C*) and coronal (*D*) T1 fat-suppressed (T1FS) images demonstrating enhancement of normal thin synovium, which extends into the popliteus tendon sheath (*arrow* in *C*) and around the cruciate ligaments (*B*, *D*).

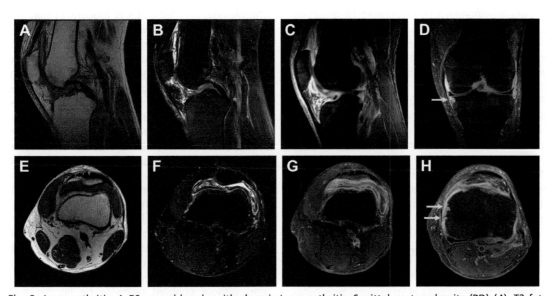

Fig. 2. Lyme arthritis. A 56-year-old male with chronic Lyme arthritis. Sagittal proton density (PD) (*A*), T2 fat-suppressed (T2FS) (*B*), postcontrast T1FS (*C*), and axial T1 (*E*), T2FS (*F*), and postcontrast T1FS (*G*) images demonstrating T1 and T2 hypointense synovial thickening with marked enhancement. Note diffuse enhancement throughout the joint with little joint effusion (*C*, *G*). Coronal (*D*) and axial postcontrast T1FS (*H*) images demonstrating erosions at the proximal medial tibia (*arrows*).

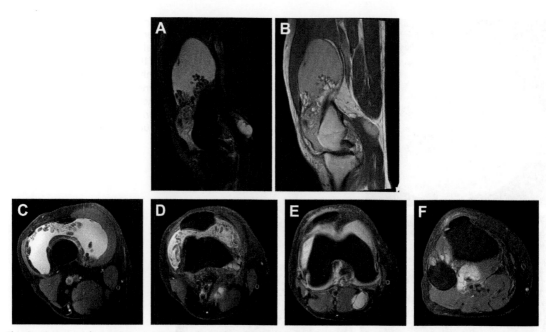

Fig. 3. Lipoma arborescens. A 57-year-old male with history of rheumatoid arthritis for 25 years, on etanercept for 15 years, with a right knee mass for 7 years. Sagittal T2FS (*A*) and T1 (*B*), and multiple axial PDFS images (*C–F*) demonstrating marked synovial proliferation and frondlike hypertrophy with a large joint effusion, which extend around the cruciate ligaments (*E*) and along the popliteus tendon sheath (*F*).

Our clinical experience is that synovitis presents as mildly hypointense synovial thickening and/or intra-articular stranding and nodularity on fluid-sensitive images. In the setting of chronic synovitis with hypertrophy of the fatty synovial villi, the villi are seen as nodular and fingerlike projections that are hypointense on fat-saturated T2-weighted and STIR images because of fat signal suppression/inversion. An extreme presentation of this finding most commonly seen in the knee is termed "lipoma arborescens," which describes a villous lipomatous proliferation of the synovium (**Fig. 3**).[15] Commonly seen in the setting of another joint pathology or insult, lipoma arborescens is theorized to be reactive in nature.[15–17] In the presence of a joint effusion, structural changes in the intra-articular fat pads have also been reported to correlate with proliferative synovitis[18,19] and may be used as a surrogate for synovitis in the absence of IV contrast, in the opinion of some authors.

POST-TRAUMATIC/OSTEOARTHRITIC SYNOVITIS

The most common cause of knee synovitis is osteoarthritis (OA). The understanding of KOA as a disease is rapidly evolving. Once thought to purely represent the manifestation of mechanical degeneration of cartilage, it later was recognized that this disorder affects the entire joint including bone, synovium, and capsule.[20] More recently, authors have proposed that OA is in fact a systemic disease with a low-grade inflammatory component particularly in obese patients.[21] Synovitis is a common finding in the setting of OA on imaging[9] and at arthroscopy.[22–24] Synovitis is thought to play an important role in the symptoms of OA[25] and its progression.[26] Innate immunity, which is the first level of immune response to inflammation, is thought to be the primary driver of synovitis in OA.[27] Pattern recognition receptors in the synovium that are supposed to be activated by microbial ligands can be stimulated by endogenous damage-associated molecular patterns that are produced by extracellular matrix damage.[28] The resulting molecular cascade results in synovitis and cartilage destruction.

Synovitis in OA is more heterogeneous and not as widespread as it is in RA.[6] Synovitis in KOA is more frequently appreciated in the suprapatellar pouch, posterior cruciate ligament recess, and the medial and lateral meniscal recesses (**Figs. 4** and **5**).[9,29] Synovitis is underestimated in OA on noncontrast imaging. The synovitis that is appreciated without contrast tends to be fibrotic and shows less histologic features of acute inflammation.[23] Static contrast-enhanced imaging more accurately defines the extent of synovitis in the knee[9,23] but dynamic enhanced imaging may be

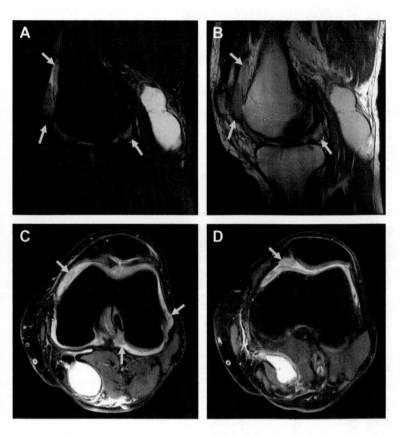

Fig. 4. Osteoarthritis. A 68-year-old male with complex medial meniscal tear and high-grade chondrosis of the medial compartment. Sagittal T2FS (*A*) and PD (*B*), and two axial PDFS images (*C*, *D*) demonstrating mildly PD and T2 hypointense synovial thickening (*arrows*) relative to joint fluid. There is also a Baker cyst seen on all of the images.

more accurate at characterizing histologically confirmed acute inflammation of synovial tissue.[30]

Other findings in KOA include subchondral cysts, bone marrow edema-like lesions, and meniscal tears/degeneration. Subchondral cysts, related to chronic overlying chondrosis, show thin peripheral enhancement because they are synovial lined. This enhancement may also appear solid if the cyst is small. Bone marrow edema-like lesions and the periphery of meniscal tears and parameniscal cysts also demonstrate enhancement.

INFLAMMATORY SYNOVITIS
Rheumatoid Arthritis

RA is an idiopathic chronic autoimmune inflammatory arthropathy affecting approximately 0.5% to 1% of the adult population.[31] Historically, physical examination and radiography were used to follow the progression of the disease. Since the introduction of disease-modifying antirheumatic drugs, MR imaging has become an indispensable tool in the evaluation of progression and treatment response, because disease findings can be subtle or beyond the sensitivity of radiographs. Although the pathogenesis of RA remains unknown, this disease's initial presentation is in the synovium. Early MR imaging and radiographic findings are that of synovitis. In fact, the presence of enhancing synovium on gadolinium-enhanced MR imaging has been described as the most common finding in the knees of patients with RA.[32] As in other arthropathies, acute RA synovitis has been described on noncontrast MR imaging as increased signal intensity of the synovium on proton density and T2-weighted sequences (**Fig. 6**).[33] On histopathology, intima cell hyperplasia, lymphocyte and plasma cell infiltration, and vascular hyperplasia/dilation have been reported as the most severe findings of synovitis. These histologic findings are distinct from that of OA. Additional findings that are appreciated on MR imaging as the disease progresses include destruction of articular and meniscal cartilage. Bony erosions are seen as areas of increased signal intensity on T2, STIR, and proton density (PD) sequences, correlating with high populations of osteoclasts and inflammatory cells on histopathology,[33] typically adjacent to the hypertrophied, hypervascular synovitis.

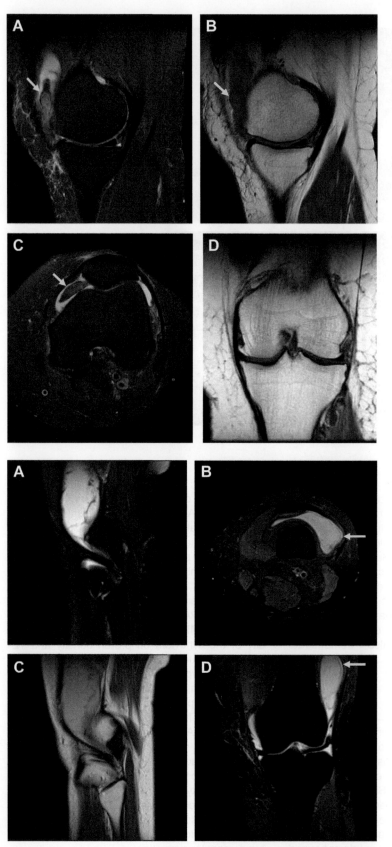

Fig. 5. Infarcted synovium. A 63-year-old female with OA and infarcted synovium mimicking a synovial mass. Sagittal T2FS (*A*) and PD (*B*), and axial T2FS demonstrating mass-like synovitis (*arrows* in *A–C*) in the anterolateral knee joint with peripheral T2 and PD hypointensity, pathologically proven to be infarcted synovium. Coronal T1-weighted image (*D*) demonstrating osteophytes.

Fig. 6. Rheumatoid arthritis. A 45-year-old female with rheumatoid arthritis and some lupus features. Sagittal T2FS (*A*), axial PDFS (*B*), sagittal PD (*C*), and coronal PDFS (*D*) demonstrate large joint effusion with mild synovitis. Note the hyperintense synovial thickening (*arrows* in *B* and *D*). This patient had only mild patellofemoral chondrosis and no internal derangement.

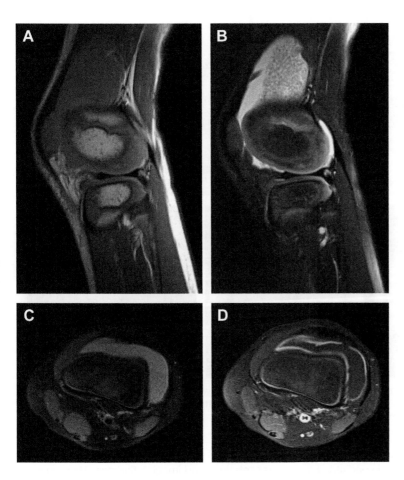

Fig. 7. JIA. A 6-year-old female with oligoarticular JIA. Sagittal PD (*A*) and T2FS (*B*), and axial PDFS (*C*) images demonstrating innumerable PD isointense-to-hypointense and T2 hypointense rice bodies and a joint effusion. Axial postcontrast T1FS (*D*) demonstrating thickened enhancing synovium.

Rice bodies, which are mildly T2 isointense to hypointense nodules[34] within the joint that resemble grains of rice, may be present. A nonspecific response to chronic synovial inflammation, rice bodies have been described in various inflammatory arthropathies and chronic infections.[35] Their exact origin is debated: whether they represent detached synovial villi[36] or infarcted synovium,[37] versus cells trapped in fibrinous joint exudate.[38] In contrast to the intra-articular cartilage fragments seen in synovial chondromatosis, which are difficult to separate from T2 hyperintense joint fluid, rice bodies are easily identified on T2-weighted images but difficult to identify on T1-weighted images (**Fig. 7**; see also **Fig. 13**).[39]

Juvenile Idiopathic Arthritis

Juvenile idiopathic arthritis (JIA), previously known as juvenile RA, is a group of arthropathies initially presenting in patients younger than age 16 years.[40] JIA is a diagnosis of exclusion and shares many clinical and imaging features with other pediatric inflammatory arthropathies. Synovial proliferation and infiltration of inflammatory cells in affected joints leads to synovial hypertrophy, joint effusion, and erosions.[40] Seven JIA subtypes are recognized: oligoarthritis, rheumatoid factor (RF) positive polyarthritis, RF negative polyarthritis, systemic arthritis, (juvenile) psoriatic arthritis, enthesitis-related arthritis, and undifferentiated arthritis.[41] The psoriatic and enthesitis-related subtypes share more clinical and imaging features with seronegative spondyloarthropathies, described in the next section. MR imaging has repeatedly been demonstrated to be superior to physical examination in the diagnosis of early JIA and is now commonly used in the work-up of suspected JIA. The early diagnosis of JIA is believed to be associated with better outcomes and a lower likelihood of long-term autoimmune inflammation and joint damage[42] when the disease is successfully treated.

The primary distinguishing imaging feature of JIA on MR imaging compared with other pediatric arthropathies is synovitis. Synovial hypertrophy

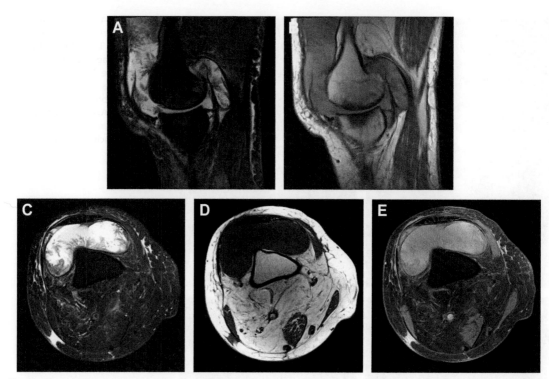

Fig. 8. Chronic JIA. A 53-year-old male with JIA presented at age 6, now with severe secondary OA. Sagittal T2FS (*A*) and PD (*B*) and axial T2FS (*C*), T1 (*D*), and PDFS (*E*) images demonstrating mildly T2 and PD hypointense and mildly T1 hyperintense synovial proliferation relative to joint fluid.

has been seen up to 61.4% of the time in patients with JIA, versus 19.4% of the time in pediatric patients with non-JIA arthropathies.[40] In the validated Juvenile Arthritis MRI Scoring system (JAMRIS), synovitis is defined as an area of synovium with increased signal that is thicker than 2 mm, averaging up to 4.8 mm (**Fig. 7**; **Fig. 8**).[43,44] In one series, the synovium homogenously enhanced on gadolinium-enhanced MR imaging in roughly half of cases versus heterogeneous enhancement in the other half, with variable signal on unenhanced T1, T2, and intermediate sequences.[43] The lack of synovitis on MR imaging in patients with clinically active disease has been shown to correlate with increased age at diagnosis and RF-negative polyarticular disease.[42] Conversely, no significant differences were found in patients with JIA versus without JIA regarding bone marrow edema or articular erosions.[40] Other common findings in JIA include joint effusion, thickening/heterogeneous signal/nodularity of Hoffa fat pad, meniscal hypoplasia, and popliteal cysts.[43]

Seronegative Spondyloarthropathies

The seronegative spondyloarthropathies are a diverse group of autoimmune inflammatory arthropathies with similar musculoskeletal clinical presentations and imaging findings. This group of disorders includes ankylosing spondylitis, reactive arthritis, psoriatic arthritis, and arthritis associated with inflammatory bowel disease. Unlike in RA, RF is typically negative. However, HLA-B27 is often positive in these conditions. Common clinical presentations include enthesitis, synovitis, spondylitis, uveitis, sacroiliitis, and inflammatory bowel disease.[44]

Enthesitis- inflammation at the attachment sites of tendons, ligaments, fascia, and joint capsules to bones- is believed to precede synovitis in most patients with SpA, and in some, may precede the onset of musculoskeletal symptoms.[45] Marrow edema in psoriatic arthritis, particularly early in the disease, is often located close to the entheses, as opposed to capsular attachments and subchondral bone in OA and RA, respectively.[44,46] Otherwise, the imaging findings of synovitis on MR imaging are like those seen in JIA and RA, particularly later in the disease (**Fig. 9**).

INFECTIOUS SYNOVITIS

Infectious arthritis can occur because of hematogenous dissemination, direct inoculation from trauma or iatrogenic sources, contiguous spread

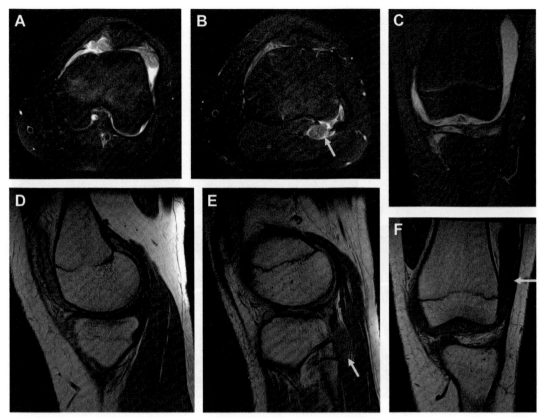

Fig. 9. Enthesitis-related arthritis. A 14-year-old female with HLA-B27-positive enthesitis-related arthritis involving her left knee. Axial PDFS (*A, B*), coronal PDFS (*C*), sagittal PD (*D, E*), and coronal T1-weighted (*F*) images demonstrating mildly PD hypointense synovial proliferation, which extends in a masslike fashion into the popliteus tendon sheath (*arrows* in *B* and *E*). Mild T1-hyperintensity of the thickened synovium (*arrow* in *F*) allows differentiation from more hypointense joint fluid.

from adjacent abscess, or adjacent osteomyelitis. Most common causes of knee suppurative arthritis include gonococcus, staphylococcus, streptococcus, *Haemophilus influenzae*, and gram-negative bacilli. The most common pathogen varies with age, with *H influenzae* predominating in children less than 2 years old, *Staphylococcus aureus* being the most common cause in children and adults, and gonococcus being prevalent in adolescence and early adulthood. Patients with sickle cell disease are prone to infection with *Salmonella* organisms at any age. The knee is the most common joint infected in nongonococcal septic arthritis.[47]

The clinical presentation of a suppurative arthritis of the knee involves acute onset of pain, a warm and swollen joint, and painful restricted range of motion. Systemic findings of fever and elevated white count are helpful, but not always present. Elevated inflammatory markers are nearly always present. On MRI, septic arthritis causes nonspecific synovitis similar to noninfectious etiologies.[48] It is a common misconception that

synovial enhancement equates with joint infection, however, thickening and enhancement of the synovium is commonly present regardless of the cause of synovitis. While MRI with and without contrast will delinate synovitis and help in the diagnosis of osteomyelitis, joint aspiration with fluid cell count and culture is required to exclude septic arthritis.[8]

If MR imaging is performed, there are a few MR imaging findings that are more likely to be seen in a septic knee compared with other causes of synovitis.[48] The presence of bone erosion, particularly when combined with diffuse bone marrow edema-like signal in the adjacent subchondral bone and enhancement of the erosion, increase the likelihood that the synovitis may be secondary to an infectious cause (see **Fig. 9**). Adjacent soft tissue abscess, sinus tract, and osteomyelitis of articular bone also increase the likelihood of septic arthritis (**Figs. 10** and **11**).

The MR imaging findings of septic arthritis including synovitis, periarticular soft tissue edema, and bone marrow edema-like signal can persist

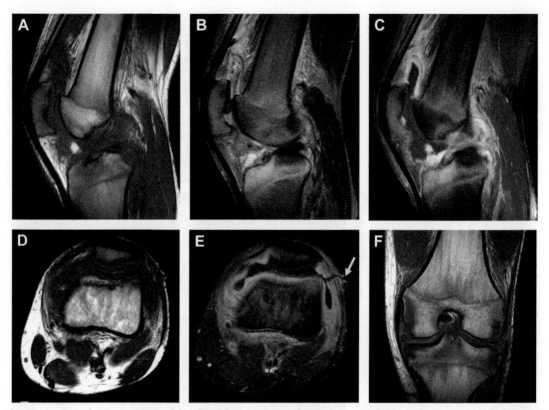

Fig. 10. Septic arthritis. A 17-year-old male with septic knee after arthroscopy for loose body. Sagittal T1 (*A*), T2FS (*B*), postcontrast T1FS (*C*), and axial T1 (*D*) and postcontrast T1FS (*E*) images demonstrating mildly T1 hyperintense and mixed T2 signal intensity synovial thickening with marked enhancement. There is extensive surrounding soft tissue edema and nonenhancing central joint fluid with arthroscopy tracks (*arrow* in *E*) through the overlying skin, consistent with intra-articular abscess and sinus tract formation. Coronal T1 (*F*) demonstrates multifocal and confluent T1 hypointense marrow signal, consistent with osteomyelitis.

despite successful treatment of the infection.[49] The presence of an abscess or a large effusion suggests incomplete eradication of an infection on post-treatment MR imaging.

Specific Organisms

Tuberculous (TB) arthritis usually results from hematogenous spread or adjacent osteomyelitis and is a chronic progressive monoarticular process. Onset is gradual with progressive pain. Over time the mycobacterium invading into the synovium causes confluent pannus formation, which may erode the bone.[47] The synovial hypertrophy in tuberculous arthritis is T2 hypointense, which may help narrow the differential. Other processes that can cause marked T2 hypointense synovial hypertrophy include gout, tenosynovial giant cell tumor, amyloidosis, and siderotic synovitis/hemophilic arthropathy,[50] discussed in the next section. Amyloidosis presents in chronic renal

failure patients, most commonly involving the hips, shoulders, and spine. Chronic gout presents as a polyarticular process, which differentiates it from tuberculous arthritis. In TB arthritis, marrow reactive change manifests as T2 hyperintensity in juxta-articular bone and there is commonly myositis present in adjacent musculature.[51] Untreated tuberculosis arthritis leads to severe destruction of the joint with fibrous ankylosis.[47]

Lyme arthritis is caused by the spirochete *Borrelia burgdorferi*, which is transmitted via a tick bite and is endemic in the northeastern United States and parts of Europe. Most patients with untreated disease manifest joint symptoms within weeks to 2 years following infection. Joint involvement tends to be remitting and migratory with one to two joints affected at a time. The knee is the most commonly affected joint.[47] Lyme arthritis causes nonspecific joint effusion and synovial hypertrophy (see **Fig. 2**; **Figs. 12** and **13**). Some authors suggest three findings that are more

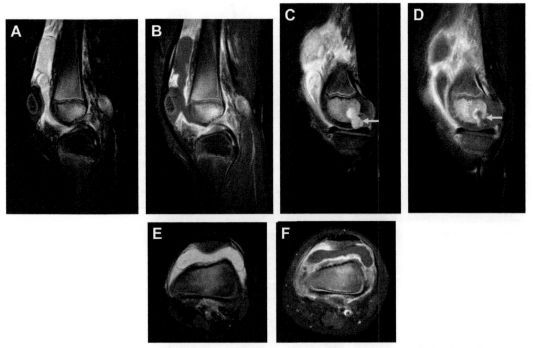

Fig. 11. Septic arthritis. A 5-year-old male with osteomyelitis and septic arthritis. Sagittal T2FS (*A* and *C*), sagittal postcontrast T1FS (*B* and *D*) and axial T2FS (*E*) and postcontrast T1FS (*F*) images demonstrating a large joint effusion with synovial thickening and enhancement. Note the extensive surrounding soft tissue edema and enhancement, with a lobulated rim-enhancing intraosseous abscess in the distal femoral epiphysis (*arrows* in *C* and *D*) with surrounding osteomyelitis.

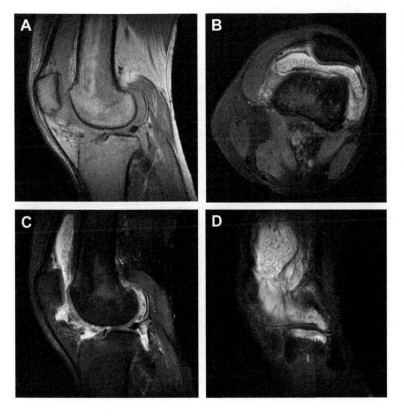

Fig. 12. Lyme arthritis. A 27-year-old male with Lyme arthritis. Sagittal PD (*A*), axial T2FS (*B*), and two sagittal T2 SPIR (*C*, *D*) images demonstrating innumerable PD isointense-to-hypointense and T2 hypointense rice bodies and a joint effusion. Note less surrounding soft tissue edema compared with bacterial septic arthritis (see **Figs. 10** and **11**).

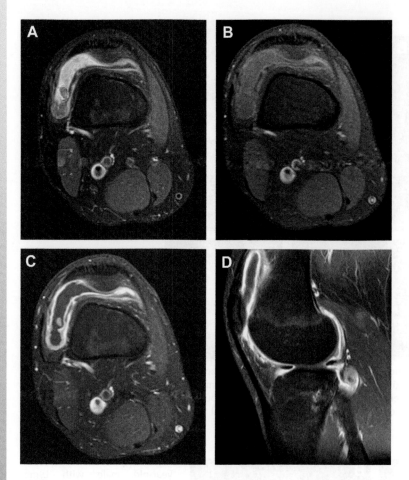

Fig. 13. Lyme arthritis. A 17-year-old male with chronic arthritis of right knee following an acute Lyme infection. Axial T2FS (*A*), T1FS (*B*), and axial (*C*) and sagittal (*D*) postcontrast T1FS images demonstrating T2 hypointense synovial thickening and nodularity, with mild intrinsic T1 hyperintensity, and marked gadolinium enhancement. Note less surrounding soft tissue edema compared with bacterial septic arthritis (see **Figs. 10 and 11**).

suggestive of Lyme arthritis rather than typical bacterial arthritis are: (1) myositis, (2) lymphadenopathy, and (3) lack of subcutaneous edema/cellulitis.[52]

Viral arthritis can occur because of parvovirus B19, rubella, and hepatitis C virus. Presentation is acute or subacute. It is unclear if the virus directly infects the synovium or if the viral infection generates an autoimmune reaction.[47] MR imaging findings of viral arthritis are nonspecific and similar to other forms of infected arthritis or reactive arthritis.

SIDEROTIC SYNOVITIS

Siderotic synovitis is seen with any process that causes recurrent bleeding into the knee joint. Common causes of siderotic synovitis include hemophilic arthropathy, tenosynovial giant cell tumor, and intra-articular vascular malformation, such as synovial hemangioma or destructive angiodysplastic arthritis. The characteristic feature of siderotic synovitis on MR imaging is

hemosiderin staining of the synovium, which manifests as marked T2 hypointensity and blooming on gradient echo imaging.[50] This finding is caused by hemosiderin deposition and signal dephasing induced by iron molecules in the synovium.

SUMMARY

Knee synovitis is a nonspecific finding seen in the setting of joint damage and inflammation, with causes ranging from post-traumatic and OA to inflammatory and infectious causes. Findings of synovial thickening, joint effusion, and synovial enhancement are present across the spectrum of etiologies and do not allow distinction. In conjunction with clinical and laboratory signs, the most specific MR imaging findings for the underlying pathology are found in the bone and adjacent soft tissues. For post-traumatic/OA, evidence of meniscal, ligamentous, and cartilage damage should be sought. Erosions are seen in inflammatory and infectious arthritides. The inflammatory arthropathies, such as RA and psoriatic arthritis, require correlation with clinical and laboratory findings. The most specific signs of acute infectious arthritis are diffuse bone marrow edema, adjacent soft tissue abscess, sinus tract, and osteomyelitis. IV contrast is helpful across the board to distinguish joint fluid from synovial proliferation and imaging should be performed in the first few minutes after injection. Delayed postcontrast imaging has been studied in various pathologies, but has not yet been shown to add value clinically.[14]

CLINICS CARE POINTS

- Knee synovitis is a nonspecific finding seen in the setting of joint damage and inflammation.
- Findings of synovial thickening, joint effusion, and synovial enhancement are present across the spectrum of etiologies and do not allow a specific diagnosis in most cases.
- The most specific signs of acute infectious arthritis are diffuse bone marrow edema, adjacent soft tissue abscess, sinus tract, and osteomyelitis.
- IV contrast is helpful to distinguish joint fluid from synovial proliferation and imaging should be performed in the first few minutes after injection.

DISCLOSURE

The authors have nothing to disclose.

REFERENCES

1. Veale D, Firestein GS. Synovium. In: Kelley and Firestein's textbook of rheumatology. 10th edition. WB Saunders; 2017. p. 20–33.
2. Goldring SR, Goldring MB. Biology of the normal joint. In: Firestein GS, Budd RC, Gabriel SE, et al, editors. Kelley and Firestein's Textbook of Rheumatology. 10th edition. WB Saunders; 2017. p. 1–19.
3. Acanfora C, Bruno F, Palumbo P, et al. Diagnostic and interventional radiology fundamentals of synovial pathology. Acta Bio Med Atenei Parm 2020; 91(Suppl 8):107.
4. Krenn V, Morawietz L, Häupl T, et al. Grading of chronic synovitis: a histopathological grading system for molecular and diagnostic pathology. Pathol Res Pract 2002;198(5):317–25.
5. Hemke R, van den Berg JM, Nusman CM, et al. Contrast-enhanced MRI findings of the knee in healthy children; establishing normal values. Eur Radiol 2018;28(3):1167.
6. Riis RGC, Gudbergsen H, Henriksen M, et al. Synovitis assessed on static and dynamic contrast-enhanced magnetic resonance imaging and its association with pain in knee osteoarthritis: a cross-sectional study. Eur J Radiol 2016;85(6): 1099–108.
7. American College of Radiology ACR Appropriateness Criteria ® Chronic Extremity Joint Pain-Suspected Inflammatory Arthritis. Available at: https://acsearch.acr.org/list. Accessed December 20, 2021.
8. American College of Radiology ACR Appropriateness Criteria ® Clinical Condition: Suspected Osteomyelitis, Septic Arthritis, or Soft Tissue Infection (Excluding Spine and Diabetic Foot). Available at: https://acsearch.acr.org/list. Accessed December 20, 2021.
9. Roemer FW, Kassim Javaid M, Guermazi A, et al. Anatomical distribution of synovitis in knee osteoarthritis and its association with joint effusion assessed on non-enhanced and contrast-enhanced MRI. Osteoarthr Cartil 2010;18(10):1269–74.
10. Hayashi D, Roemer F, Guermazi A. Imaging for osteoarthritis. Ann Phys Rehabil Med 2016;59(3):161–9.
11. Guermazi A, Roemer F, Hayashi D, et al. Assessment of synovitis with contrast-enhanced MRI using a whole-joint semiquantitative scoring system in people with, or at high risk of, knee osteoarthritis: the MOST study. Ann Rheum Dis 2011;70(5):805–11.
12. Singson RD, Zalduondo FM. Value of unenhanced spin-echo MR imaging in distinguishing between synovitis and effusion of the knee. Am J Roentgenol 1992;159(3):569–71.
13. Beltran J, Caudill JL, Herman LA, et al. Rheumatoid arthritis: MR imaging manifestations. Radiology 1987;165(1):153–7.
14. Bjorkcngren AG, Geborek P, Rydholm U, et al. MR imaging of the knee in acute rheumatoid arthritis: synovial uptake of gadolinium-DOTA. Am J Roentgenol 1990;155(2):329–32.
15. Feller J, Rishi M, Hughes E. Lipoma arborescens of the knee: MR demonstration. Am J Roentgenol 1994;163(1):162–4.
16. Grieten M, Buckwalter K, Cardinal E, et al. Case report 873: lipoma arborescens (villous lipomatous proliferation of the synovial membrane). Skeletal Radiol 1994;23(8):652–5.
17. Dawson J, Dowling F, Preston B, et al. Case report: lipoma arborescens of the sub-deltoid bursa. Br J Radiol 1995;68(806):197–9.
18. Schweitzer ME, Falk A, Pathria M, et al. MR imaging of the knee: can changes in the intracapsular fat pads be used as a sign of synovial proliferation in the presence of an effusion? Am J Roentgenol 1993;160(4):823–6.

19. Roemer FW, Guermazi A, Zhang Y, et al. Hoffa's fat pad: evaluation on unenhanced MR images as a measure of patellofemoral synovitis in osteoarthritis. Am J Roentgenol 2009;192(6):1696–700.

20. Loeser R, Goldring S, Scanzello C, et al. Osteoarthritis: a disease of the joint as an organ. Arthritis Rheum 2012;64(6):1697–707.

21. Wang T, He C. Pro-inflammatory cytokines: the link between obesity and osteoarthritis. Cytokine Growth Factor Rev 2018;44:38–50.

22. Fernandez-Madrid F, Karvonen R, Teitge R, et al. Synovial thickening detected by MR imaging in osteoarthritis of the knee confirmed by biopsy as synovitis. Magn Reson Imaging 1995;13(2):177–83.

23. Loeuille D, Sauliere N, Champigneulle J, et al. Comparing non-enhanced and enhanced sequences in the assessment of effusion and synovitis in knee OA: associations with clinical, macroscopic and microscopic features. Osteoarthr Cartil 2011;19(12):1433–9.

24. Liu L, Ishijima M, Futami I, et al. Correlation between synovitis detected on enhanced-magnetic resonance imaging and a histological analysis with a patient-oriented outcome measure for Japanese patients with end-stage knee osteoarthritis receiving joint replacement surgery. Clin Rheumatol 2010;29(10):1185–90.

25. Baker K, Grainger A, Niu J, et al. Relation of synovitis to knee pain using contrast-enhanced MRIs. Ann Rheum Dis 2010;69(10):1779–83.

26. Roemer F, Guermazi A, Felson D, et al. Presence of MRI-detected joint effusion and synovitis increases the risk of cartilage loss in knees without osteoarthritis at 30-month follow-up: the MOST study. Ann Rheum Dis 2011;70(10):1804–9.

27. Scanzello C, Plaas A, Crow M. Innate immune system activation in osteoarthritis: is osteoarthritis a chronic wound? Curr Opin Rheumatol 2008;20(5):565–72.

28. Piccinini AM, Midwood KS. DAMPening inflammation by modulating TLR signalling. Mediators Inflamm 2010;2010. https://doi.org/10.1155/2010/672395.

29. Scanzello C, McKeon B, Swaim B, et al. Synovial inflammation in patients undergoing arthroscopic meniscectomy: molecular characterization and relationship to symptoms. Arthritis Rheum 2011;63(2):391–400.

30. Shakoor D, Demehri S, Roemer F, et al. Are contrast-enhanced and non-contrast MRI findings reflecting synovial inflammation in knee osteoarthritis: a meta-analysis of observational studies. Osteoarthr Cartil 2020;28(2):126–36.

31. Gabriel S. The epidemiology of rheumatoid arthritis. Rheum Dis Clin North Am 2001;27(2):269–81.

32. Forslind K, Larsson E, Eberhardt K, et al. Magnetic resonance imaging of the knee: a tool for prediction of joint damage in early rheumatoid arthritis? Scand J Rheumatol 2004;33(3):154–61.

33. Meng X, Wang Z, Zhang X, et al. Rheumatoid arthritis of knee joints: MRI-pathological correlation. Orthop Surg 2018;10(3):247–54.

34. Griffith J, Peh W, Evans N, et al. Multiple rice body formation in chronic subacromial/subdeltoid bursitis: MR appearances. Clin Radiol 1996;51(7):511–4.

35. Chung C, Coley BD, Martin LC. Case report rice bodies in juvenile rheumatoid arthritis. AJR 1998;170(3):698–700.

36. Berg E, Wainwright R, Barton B, et al. On the nature of rheumatoid rice bodies: an immunologic, histochemical, and electron microscope study. Arthritis Rheum 1977;20(7):1343–9.

37. Cheung H, Ryan L, Kozin F, et al. Synovial origins of rice bodies in joint fluid. Arthritis Rheum 1980;23(1):72–6.

38. Gálvez J, Sola J, Ortuño G, et al. Microscopic rice bodies in rheumatoid synovial fluid sediments. J Rheumatol 1992;19(12):1851–8.

39. Chen A, Wong L-Y, Sheu C-Y, et al. Distinguishing multiple rice body formation in chronic subacromial-subdeltoid bursitis from synovial chondromatosis. Skeletal Radiol 2001 312 2001;31(2):119–21.

40. Hemke R, Kuijpers TW, Nusman CM, et al. Contrast-enhanced MRI features in the early diagnosis of juvenile idiopathic arthritis. Eur Radiol 2015;25(11):3222.

41. Petty R, Southwood T, Manners P, et al. International League of Associations for Rheumatology classification of juvenile idiopathic arthritis: second revision, Edmonton, 2001. J Rheumatol 2004;31(2):390–2. https://www.jrheum.org/content/jrheum/31/2/390.full.pdf.

42. van Gulik E, Hemke R, Welsink-Karssies M, et al. Normal MRI findings of the knee in patients with clinically active juvenile idiopathic arthritis. Eur J Radiol 2018;102:36–40.

43. Gylys-Morin V, Graham T, Blebea J, et al. Knee in early juvenile rheumatoid arthritis: MR imaging findings. Radiology 2001;220(3):696–706.

44. Yasser R, Yasser E, Hanan D, et al. Enthesitis in seronegative spondyloarthropathies with special attention to the knee joint by MRI: a step forward toward understanding disease pathogenesis. Clin Rheumatol 2011;30(3):313–22.

45. Emad Y, Ragab Y, Gheita T, et al. Knee enthesitis and synovitis on magnetic resonance imaging in patients with psoriasis without arthritic symptoms. J Rheumatol 2012;39(10):1979–86.

46. Mathew A, Østergaard M. Magnetic resonance imaging of enthesitis in spondyloarthritis, including psoriatic arthritis: status and recent advances. Front Med 2020;7. https://doi.org/10.3389/FMED.2020.00296.

47. Kumar V, Abbas AK, Fausto N, et al. Robbins and Cotran pathologic basis of disease. 7th edition. Elsevier Saunders; 2005.

48. Graif M, Schweitzer M, Deely D, et al. The septic versus nonseptic inflamed joint: MRI characteristics. Skeletal Radiol 1999;28(11):616–20.

49. Bierry G, Huang A, Chang C, et al. MRI findings of treated bacterial septic arthritis. Skeletal Radiol 2012;41(12):1509–16.

50. Narváez J, Narváez J, Ortega R, et al. Hypointense synovial lesions on T2-weighted images: differential diagnosis with pathologic correlation. AJR Am J Roentgenol 2003;181(3):761–9.

51. Sanghvi DA, Iyer VR, Deshmukh T, et al. MRI features of tuberculosis of the knee. Skelet Radiol 2008;38(3):267–73.

52. Ecklund K, Vargas S, Zurakowski D, et al. MRI features of Lyme arthritis in children. AJR Am J Roentgenol 2012;184(6):1904–9.

Knee Plical Pathology and Impingement Syndromes

Megan K. Mills, MD*, Hailey Allen, MD

KEYWORDS

- Plica • Impingement syndromes • Knee • Friction syndromes • Snapping tendon

KEY POINTS

- Discuss plica anatomy, pathophysiology, and treatment
- Describe common impingement syndromes about the knee
- Review the imaging findings associated with common impingement syndromes and plical pathology about the knee

INTRODUCTION

MR imaging is a key tool in the diagnostic evaluation of patients with chronic knee pain. Although less common than osteoarthritis, ligamentous, or meniscal pathology, it is important to recognize imaging manifestations of painful impingement syndromes because such findings can explain patient symptoms and guide appropriate management. Impingement syndromes are caused by anatomic variability of normal structures, altered biomechanics, or a combination of both.

This article reviews the normal and abnormal imaging appearance of structures implicated in impingement syndromes including synovial plicae, intracapsular fat pads, and the iliotibial band (ITB). Anatomic features that may predispose to symptoms, impingement pathophysiology, and the basics of clinical management are discussed.

KNEE PLICAE
Plica Embryology and Histology

Synovial plicae are believed to represent remnant septations from the embryonic stage of knee development in which mesodermal elements condense to form medial, lateral, and patellofemoral compartments separated by synovial membranes.[1] The synovial barriers separating the compartments fuse together and resorb late within the first trimester of pregnancy; the plicae seen in adult patients represent sites of incomplete resorption of those septations.[1]

Normal synovial plicae are thin, pliable structures that can appear nearly transparent on arthroscopy. Histologically, plicae are composed of dense connective tissue containing collagen and small blood vessels. Although plicae are sometimes described qualitatively as being "elastic," histologic studies show that elastin fibers within the plicae are rare.[2] Small peripheral nerves have been found at the margin of the infrapatellar plica and Hoffa fat pad.[3] Normal plicae are thin, hypointense, bandlike structures on MR imaging with preserved signal of their adjacent fat pads. Because normal plicae are extremely common and are not associated with patient symptoms, they are frequently and prudently not mentioned on MR imaging reports.[4]

Plica Morphology

Infrapatellar plica

The infrapatellar plica is the most commonly encountered plica at arthroscopy, seen in 85% of patients.[5] It is located midline within the anterior inferior joint space, arising as a narrow band from the intercondylar notch and coursing inferiorly/anteriorly to blend with Hoffa fat pad. It may adhere to the anterior margin of the anterior

Department of Radiology & Imaging Sciences, University of Utah School of Medicine, 30 North 1900 East #1A071, Salt Lake City, UT 84132-2140, USA
* Corresponding author.
E-mail address: Megan.Mills@hsc.utah.edu

Magn Reson Imaging Clin N Am 30 (2022) 293–305
https://doi.org/10.1016/j.mric.2021.11.008
1064-9689/22/Published by Elsevier Inc.

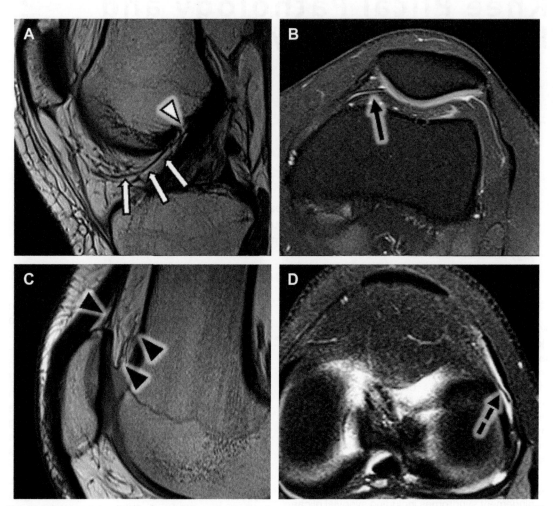

Fig. 1. MR images acquired in four adult patients showing normal synovial plicae. (*A*) Sagittal proton density (PD) image demonstrating a normal infrapatellar plica (*arrows*) as a thin hypointense band arising from the intercondylar notch and inserting on the posterior aspect of Hoffa fat pad. This plica shows an attachment to the ACL (*arrowhead*), consistent with a vertical septum type plica. (*B*) Axial PD fat-suppressed image showing a normal medial patellar plica (*arrow*) coursing between the deep margin of the vastus medialis obliquus and Hoffa fat pad within the medial anterior knee joint. This example is shelflike and partially covers the medial femoral condyle consistent with a Sakakibara type C plica. (*C*) Sagittal PD image of a normal suprapatellar plica (*arrowheads*) forming a thin septum between the anterior femoral metaphysis and the deep quadriceps tendon (Deutsch type A/Zidorn type I). (*D*) Axial PD fat-suppressed image of a normal lateral patellar plica (*dashed arrow*), which takes a coronal oblique course from the lateral joint capsule above the popliteal hiatus to the posterior margin of Hoffa fat pad.

cruciate ligament (ACL) (**Fig. 1**).[6] In 90% of patients with an infrapatellar plica there is a small synovium-lined recess located inferior to the plica known as the ligamentum mucosum recess or the horizontal cleft of Hoffa fat pad. This recess communicates with the joint and may contain fluid, intra-articular bodies, or synovitis.[7]

Kim and colleagues[6] proposed a classification system based on infrapatellar plical morphology at arthroscopy (**Table 1**). In 60.5% of patients the plica has no attachment to the ACL; this is termed the separate type. A split type plica shows no attachment to the ACL and is split along its longitudinal axis; this is seen in 13.5% of patients. In 10.5% of patients the plica forms a complete septum, continuous with the ACL, which divides the anterior knee into medial and lateral compartments; this is termed the vertical septum type. A vertical septum type plica with a superimposed central opening is called fenestra type, seen in only 1% of patients. In 14.5% of patients no appreciable plica is seen; this is called absent type. The plica may also attach to the anterior horn of the lateral meniscus or the transverse intermeniscal ligament.[8]

Table 1 Classification systems of the infrapatellar, medial patellar, and suprapatellar plicae		
Plica Classification		
Infrapatellar Plica Classification	**Medial Patellar Plica: Sakakibara Classification**	**Suprapatellar Plica: Deutsch and Zidorn Classifications**
Separate type No attachment to the ACL	Type A Thin, cordlike Unlikely to cause symptoms	Deutsch A/Zidorn I Complete septum isolating the suprapatellar recess from the rest of the joint
Split type No attachment to the ACL, split longitudinally	Type B Small, shelflike Unlikely to cause symptoms	Deutsch B/Zidorn II Septum with central perforation
Vertical septum type Complete septum attached to the ACL	Type C Large, shelflike, covers the anterior medial femoral condyle Most likely to cause symptoms	Deutsch C/Zidorn III Incomplete, crescent-shaped septum arising from the medial quadriceps tendon
Fenestra type Septum attached to the ACL with a central opening	Type D Large, shelflike, with central fenestration Rare; may cause symptoms because of size	Zidorn IV No detectable plica
Absent type No detectable plica		

Medial patellar plica

A medial patellar plica is present in 18.5% to 80% of patients, making it the second most common plica after the infrapatellar plica.[5] It is the most likely to become symptomatic. Superiorly the medial patellar plica arises from the medial joint space along the deep margin of the vastus medialis obliquus. Inferiorly it attaches along the deep border of Hoffa fat pad (see **Fig. 1**). The Sakakibara classification describes the plica based on size and morphology (see **Table 1**).[9] A type A plica is described as thin and cordlike. A type B plica is small, shelflike, and does not significantly cover the anterior surface of the medial femoral condyle. A type C plica is large, shelflike, and covers the medial femoral condyle. The rare type D plica is large with central fenestrations. Because of their small size, types A and B are unlikely to develop symptoms, whereas the larger types C and D are more likely to become symptomatic.

Suprapatellar plica

The suprapatellar plica originates from the deep distal margin of the quadriceps tendon. It courses posterior to the suprapatellar fat pad and attaches along the medial suprapatellar pouch where it may blend with the medial patellar plica.[10] It forms a membrane between the suprapatellar recess and the rest of the knee joint that varies in size and

extent, as described by Deutsch and colleagues[11] (see **Fig. 1** and **Table 1**). A type A plica forms a complete septum separating the suprapatellar recess from the remainder of the joint; this type of plica may complicate diagnostic knee arthrography or therapeutic joint injections. A type B plica is an incomplete septum with a central perforation that allows communication between the suprapatellar recess and the joint. This type may result in intra-articular bodies passing through the perforation and becoming sequestered within the suprapatellar recess. A type C plica is incomplete, crescent-shaped, and arises from the medial quadriceps tendon. The Zidorn classification mirrors that of Deutsch, with Deutsch types A, B, and C corresponding to Zidorn types I, II, and III. Zidorn adds a type IV, which is complete absence of the plica.[11,12] The incidence of the suprapatellar plica is reported at 9.1% to 55% (see **Table 1**).[5,10,13]

Lateral patellar plica

The lateral patellar plica is the least common, at 1% to 3% reported prevalence, and is least likely to result in symptoms.[14] It lies in an oblique coronal plane, arising from the superolateral joint capsule above the popliteus hiatus and inserting on Hoffa fat pad (see **Fig. 1**).

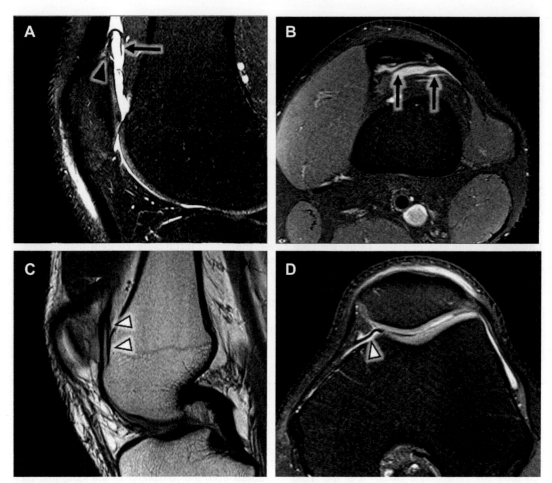

Fig. 2. A 40-year-old woman with chronic knee pain and locking. Sagittal T2-weighted fat-suppressed (*A*) and axial PD fat-suppressed (*B*) MR images show a conspicuous, mildly thickened suprapatellar plica (*arrows*). The posterior margin of the adjacent suprapatellar fat pad is mildly edematous (*arrowhead*). Sagittal PD (*C*) and axial PD fat-suppressed (*D*) MR images show an abnormally thickened medial patellar plica in the same patient (*arrowheads*).

Plica Syndrome

Although most synovial plicae remain asymptomatic, direct trauma, overuse, and intra-articular inflammatory conditions can lead to plical edema, thickening, and fibrosis. Such structural abnormalities can lead to pain and functional impairment, known as the plica syndrome. The syndrome most commonly effects young patients who participate in activities involving repetitive knee flexion and extension.[5] The medial patellar plica is most frequently implicated. The clinical presentation of plica syndrome varies and can include vague knee pain, locking, crepitation, localized tenderness, and even audible snapping. Symptoms may be limited to provoking activities or may be present at rest. Physical examination findings may include a joint effusion or crepitus. Rarely a painful palpable cord along the medial knee may be detected. Signs and symptoms can mimic meniscal tears, osteochondral lesions, and other knee impingement syndromes.[5,14] MR imaging of early or acute plica syndrome shows thickening of the plica with increased signal intensity on fluid-sensitive sequences (**Fig. 2**). There may be edema of adjacent fat pads and/or a joint effusion. At arthroscopy the plica is thickened and hypervascular. Long-standing irritation can result in marked plical thickening and fibrosis. The plica appears enlarged and hypointense on MR imaging, with or without edema of adjacent fat pads. Arthroscopically the chronically irritated plica is thick, immobile, and with irregular/frayed margins (**Figs. 3** and **4**). The medial patellar plica can be impinged between the medial patella and the

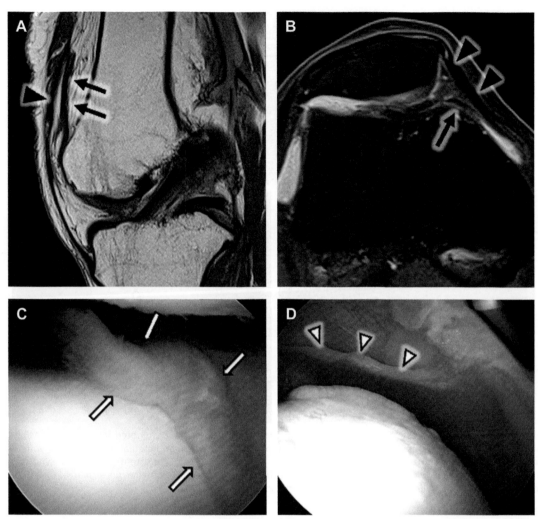

Fig. 3. A 57-year-old woman with knee pain and catching with activity. Sagittal PD (*A*) and axial PD fat-suppressed (*B*) MR images show a thickened, hyperintense medial patellar plica (*arrows*) located deep to the medial patellofemoral retinaculum (*arrowheads*). Intraoperative arthroscopic images (*C, D*) confirm an enlarged medial patellar plica (*arrows*); this was surgically resected (*arrowheads*).

anteromedial femoral condyle, which may result in chondromalacia, cartilage loss, and edema/cystic changes of the subchondral bone.[5,14,15] Chronic irritation of the infrapatellar plica may be an associated finding in Hoffa disease.[16]

Accurate diagnosis of plica syndrome is challenging because of its nonspecific signs and symptoms. If evidence of an abnormal plica is present on MR imaging and no other finding better explains the patient's presentation, plica syndrome is proposed as a cause of the patient's pain. The diagnosis relies heavily on clinical features, because not all plica that are abnormal on imaging are accompanied by symptoms of plica syndrome.

Once diagnosed, patients with plica syndrome are first managed conservatively with rest from exacerbating activities, anti-inflammatory medications, stretching/physical therapy, and localized cold or heat therapy. Intra-articular injection of anesthetics and/or corticosteroids may be performed.[17] Short duration of symptoms, young patient age, and a history of trauma predict better response to conservative treatment, although complete resolution of symptoms with such measures is rare.[18] Patients that fail to respond to nonsurgical options proceed to diagnostic arthroscopy followed by complete excision of the plica. Outcomes following plica resection are generally good with low rates of complications or plica recurrence.[15,18] Response to surgery may be better in patients with preserved articular cartilage as opposed to those with chondromalacia.[5]

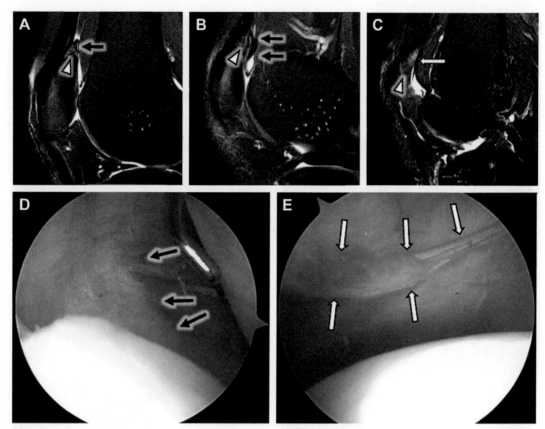

Fig. 4. A 44-year-old male ultrarunner with knee pain and stiffness. Sagittal T2-weighted fat-suppressed MR images (*A–C*) show an abnormally thickened suprapatellar plica (*black arrows*) and medial patellar plica (*white arrow*) with edema of the adjacent suprapatellar fat pad (*arrowheads*) consistent with plica syndrome. Intraoperative arthroscopic images (*D, E*) show a hypertrophied, frayed suprapatellar plica (*black arrows*) and medial patellar plica (*white arrows*), which were arthroscopically resected.

IMPINGEMENT SYNDROMES
Fat Pad Impingement

Patellofemoral pain syndrome (PFPS) is a clinically challenging and common cause of anterior knee pain in young adults. PFPS is thought to be a chronic overuse injury characterized by abnormal biomechanics including patellar maltracking or patellar malalignment, which results in injury to

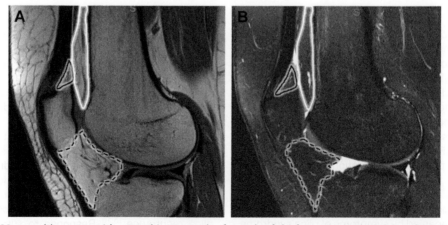

Fig. 5. A 20-year-old woman with normal intracapsular fat pads of the knee. Sagittal PD (*A*) and sagittal PD fat-suppressed (*B*) MR images of the normal quadriceps or anterior suprapatellar fat pad (*black outline*), prefemoral or posterior suprapatellar fat pad (*white outline*), and Hoffa or infrapatellar fat pad (*dashed outline*).

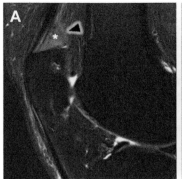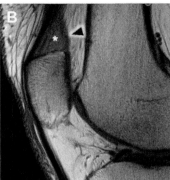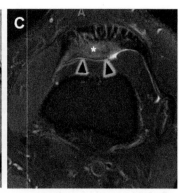

Fig. 6. A 55-year-old woman with insidious onset of knee pain localized to the superior patella. Sagittal PD fat-suppressed (*A*), sagittal PD (*B*), and axial PD fat-suppressed (*C*) MR images show increased signal and edema of the quadriceps fat pad (*asterisks*). The fat pad is enlarged with posterior bowing (*arrowheads*) into the suprapatellar joint recess consistent with quadriceps fat pad impingement.

the anterior knee osseous or soft tissue structures. Although the pathophysiology of PFPS is not well understood, one potential pain generator is impingement of the fat pads of the knee.[19]

The knee fat pads include the quadriceps (anterior suprapatellar), prefemoral (posterior suprapatellar), and Hoffa (infrapatellar) (**Fig. 5**). The fat pads are interposed between the joint capsule and the synovium with multiple sites of attachment. They are dynamic structures vital to supporting the motion of the tendons, ligaments, and osseous structures of the knee.[20,21]

Treatment of fat pat impingement is usually conservative and may include patellar taping, physical therapy, activity modification, and anti-inflammatory medication. Surgery is uncommon but may be pursued if a specific surgically correctable cause for PFPS is identified or if conservative management fails.[19]

Quadriceps fat pad impingement

The quadriceps or anterior suprapatellar fat pad is triangular and located posterior to the quadriceps tendon, anterior to the suprapatellar synovium, and superior to the patella. Injury to the suprapatellar fat pad is thought to be secondary to chronic overuse resulting in edema and hemorrhage as opposed to true impingement between adjacent structures.[22,23]

MR imaging findings of suprapatellar fat pad impingement include posterior bowing of the fat pad with mass effect on the suprapatellar joint recess and increased signal intensity on fluid-sensitive sequences (**Fig. 6**). Diagnosticians should be wary of these imaging findings in isolation or in cases of disparate clinical symptomatology. Enlargement and edema of the suprapatellar fat pad is a frequently encountered finding on knee MR imaging in asymptomatic populations.[24] In

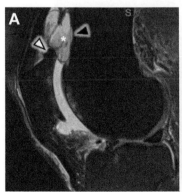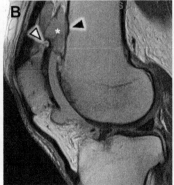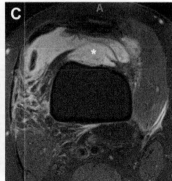

Fig. 7. A 57-year-old woman with anterior knee pain and difficulty with knee extension. Sagittal PD fat-suppressed (*A*), sagittal PD (*B*), and axial PD fat-suppressed (*C*) MR images show increased signal and enlargement of the prefemoral fat pad (*asterisks*). Note severe patellofemoral osteoarthritis and superior osteophyte (*white arrowheads*) with mechanical erosion/scalloping of the anterior distal femur (*black arrowheads*) consistent with prefemoral fat pad impingement syndrome.

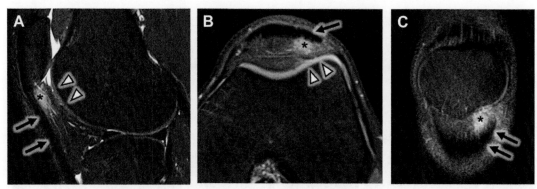

Fig. 8. A 22-year-old female cross-country runner with chronic lateral knee pain. Sagittal T2-weighted fat-suppressed (*A*), axial PD fat-suppressed (*B*), and coronal PD fat-suppressed (*C*) MR images show localized edema within the superolateral aspect of Hoffa fat pad (*asterisks*). The edema lies deep to the lateral patellar tendon (*arrows*) and superficial to the lateral femoral condyle (*arrowheads*). Findings support a diagnosis of Hoffa fat pad impingement caused by patellar tendon lateral femoral condyle friction syndrome.

one study of 879 knee MR exams, 13.8% of cases showed mass effect of the suprapatellar fat pad on the suprapatellar recess. Despite the high frequency of mass effect, only six patients in this cohort had anterior knee pain.[25]

Prefemoral fat pad impingement

The prefemoral or posterior suprapatellar fat pad is ellipsoid and is located anterior to the distal femoral metadiaphysis and posterior to the suprapatellar synovium. Prefemoral fat pad impingement syndrome (PFIS) is caused by abnormalities of the fat pad and/or the surrounding structures. Extrinsic mass effect is seen in patients with patellar tendon lateral femoral condyle friction syndrome (PT-LFCFS), other patellar maltracking abnormalities,

or is caused by prominent patellar osteophytes.[22] Primary fat pad hyperplasia or tumoral lesions, such as lipoma arborescens or lipoma, may predispose to impingement because of the increased fat pad volume.[26]

MR imaging findings in PFIS include increased signal within the fat pad on fluid-sensitive sequences and abnormal fat pad morphology. In cases of osteophytic impingement, the fat pad may be distorted or atrophic immediately adjacent to the osteophyte (**Fig. 7**).[22] Enlargement of the prefemoral fat pad should prompt additional evaluation for underlying mass because appropriate treatment may be surgical as in cases of lipoma or lipoma arborescens.[27] Similar to quadriceps fat pad impingement, imaging findings of PFIS

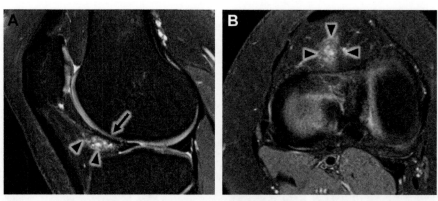

Fig. 9. A 24-year-old woman with months of anterior knee pain and clinical features of patellofemoral pain syndrome. Sagittal T2-weighted fat-suppressed (*A*) and axial PD fat-suppressed (*B*) MR images show a focus of masslike increased T2/PD signal intensity within the inferolateral aspect of Hoffa fat pad (*arrowheads*). There is thickening of the adjacent infrapatellar plica (*arrow*). Imaging findings are suggestive of acute changes of Hoffa disease with edema signal within the fat pad. Chronic impingement results in fibrosis, scarring, and eventual ossification, not yet present in this case.

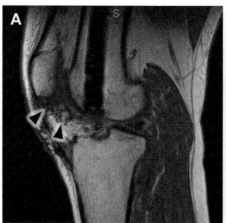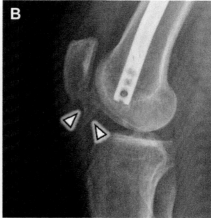

Fig. 10. A 23-year-old man with stiffness and locking of the knee in the setting of prior intramedullary nail fixation of a femoral diaphyseal fracture. Sagittal PD MR image (*A*) and lateral radiograph of the knee (*B*) show heterogenous PD signal within the superior aspect of Hoffa fat pad (*black arrowheads*) with corresponding ossification (*white arrowheads*) suggestive of chronic Hoffa disease caused by iatrogenic trauma from remote femoral fixation.

should be correlated with patient symptoms because edema of the prefemoral fat pad was seen in 19% of knee MR exams in one asymptomatic study population.[28]

Hoffa Fat Pad Impingement

The Hoffa or infrapatellar fat pad is rectangular and is located inferior to the patella, posterior to the patellar tendon, anterior to the infrapatellar synovium, and superior to the proximal tibia. The anatomy and function of Hoffa fat pad is complex with multiple septations, robust innervation, internal plica, and an important role in biomechanical function.[29]

Three types of Hoffa fat pad impingement have been described: (1) impingement in PT-LFCFS, (2) infrapatellar plica impingement, and (3) Hoffa disease. PT-LFCFS is an overuse injury because of repetitive compression of Hoffa fat pad between the patellar tendon and lateral femoral condyle. Patients present with typical symptoms of PFPS and anterior knee pain that can mimic patellar tendonitis. Patellar maltracking may play a role in this disease process, with one study demonstrating patella alta or lateral patellar subluxation in 33/42 and 4/42 patients with PT-LFCFS, respectively.[30] Imaging findings of PT-LFCFS include increased signal on fluid-sensitive sequences in the superolateral aspect of Hoffa fat pad, deep

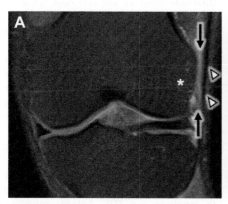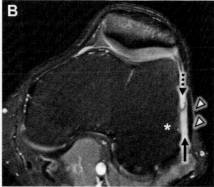

Fig. 11. A 35-year-old man presenting with anterior knee pain while training for a marathon. Coronal (*A*) and axial (*B*) PD fat-suppressed images show increased fluid signal and edema (*arrows*) deep to the ITB (*arrowheads*) and superficial to the lateral femoral epicondyle (*asterisks*), consistent with ITB friction syndrome. Note the edema is separate and posterior to the normal superolateral joint recess (*dashed arrow*). ITB friction syndrome is misdiagnosed if the normal superolateral joint recess is mistaken for pathologic edema/fluid.

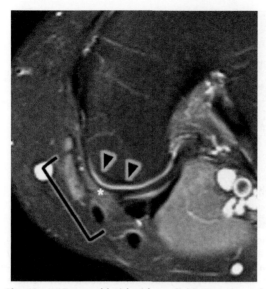

Fig. 12. A 15-year-old girl with medial knee pain and mechanical symptoms exacerbated by running. Axial PD fat-suppressed MR image shows focal edema (*asterisk*) within the soft tissues deep to the sartorius and gracilis tendons (*bracket*) and superficial to the posteromedial femoral condyle (*arrowheads*). Findings were suggestive of posteromedial knee friction syndrome.

to the lateral patellar tendon and superficial to the lateral femoral condyle (**Fig. 8**).

A related but distinct entity is Hoffa disease. This process is the result of acute trauma or chronic repetitive injury to Hoffa fat pad resulting in hemorrhage. The fat pad can become hypertrophied, predisposing to further impingement and a cycle of injury.[31] In acute cases, edema and hemorrhage predominate, whereas chronic cases present with fibrosis and scarring. On MR imaging, acute Hoffa disease has increased signal within the fat pad on fluid-sensitive sequences. Heterogenous morphology and signal intensity is seen because of hemorrhage (**Fig. 9**). In chronic cases, fibrosis and hemosiderin deposition result in decreased MR imaging signal on all sequences. Eventual ossification of the fat pad may occur (**Fig. 10**).

Tendon Impingement and Friction Syndromes

Several soft tissue structures about the knee are predisposed to chronic irritation from repetitive motion, most notably the tendons and adjacent soft tissues. Because of the complex joint motion and number of structures in a confined space, changes in biomechanics or activity levels can result in pain and pathology. These disease processes have been described as impingement, friction, and snapping syndromes.

Iliotibial band friction syndrome

ITB friction syndrome is thought to be the most common impingement syndrome about the knee. This chronic repetitive injury occurs as the ITB moves over the lateral femoral epicondyle during knee flexion and extension. The ITB is taut in extension and lies immediately anterior to the lateral femoral epicondyle. During knee flexion the ITB translates posterior, over the lateral femoral epicondyle, and superficial to the posterior lateral corner structures. Repetitive knee flexion and extension can cause an inflammatory response in the fat and soft tissues that reside deep to the ITB and superficial to the lateral femoral epicondyle. Biomechanical factors, such as genu varum or abnormal foot pronation, may further predispose to ITB impingement by increasing ITB tension and/or narrowing the space between the ITB, femoral condyle, and posterior lateral corner structures. The anteroposterior diameter or thickness of the ITB may play a role in impingement in some patients, with an increased incidence of ITB friction syndrome in running athletes who had an increased ITB diameter.[32]

Patients with ITB friction syndrome are usually long-distance runners or cyclists, often those reporting a recent increase in activity. The clinical presentation includes pain with palpation of the lateral femoral epicondyle and reproduction of symptoms with active or passive knee flexion/extension. Intra-articular pathology, such as lateral meniscus tears or fibular collateral ligament injuries, can have a similar clinical presentation to ITB friction syndrome. In such cases, imaging plays a vital role in making a diagnosis.

MR imaging findings of ITB friction syndrome include increased signal on fluid-sensitive sequences deep to the ITB and superficial to the lateral femoral epicondyle. Patients may have edema of the involved soft tissues or a fluid collection/adventitial bursa.[33,34] An imaging pitfall in diagnosing ITB friction syndrome is misidentification of normal joint fluid within the lateral synovial recess as pathologic fluid. The lateral synovial recess should be identified immediately anterior to the lateral femoral epicondyle, whereas fluid in ITB friction syndrome should be located lateral or posterior to the lateral femoral epicondyle (**Fig. 11**).

Treatment of ITB friction syndrome is typically conservative with emphasis on stretching/rolling to lengthen the ITB. Activity modification and anti-inflammatory medication may be used as needed. If conservative treatment fails to resolve symptoms, anesthetic or corticosteroid injection may be used. Surgical release of the ITB is

Table 2
Impingement syndromes of knee by anatomic location

Impingement Syndromes of the Knee			
Anatomic Location	Anterior Compartment	Medial Compartment	Lateral Compartment
Extracapsular		Posteromedial knee friction syndrome	Iliotibial band friction syndrome
Intracapsular	Quadriceps fat pad impingement Prefemoral fat pad impingement Hoffa fat pad impingement Suprapatellar plica impingement	Medial plica syndrome	Popliteus tendon impingement

indicated in rare cases. Predisposing deformities, such as genu varum, may require specific treatment to fully address ITB friction syndrome.

Posteromedial knee friction syndrome

A friction syndrome in the posteromedial knee has been recently described and is thought to result from a narrowed space between the sartorius and gracilis tendons and the adjacent posterior medial femoral condyle.[35] Narrowing of the space results in chronic irritation of the intervening fat during knee flexion and extension. Patients with posteromedial knee friction syndrome present with medial joint line pain, which can mimic other intra-articular disease processes. In a study by Simeone and colleagues,[35] 42% of subjects with posteromedial knee friction were initially clinically suspected to have a medial meniscus tear. MR imaging plays a vital role in distinguishing these two conditions that have different management. MR imaging findings of posteromedial knee friction include edema of the fat interposed between the medial femoral condyle and the sartorius and/or gracilis tendons, often with a narrowed space (**Fig. 12**). Osseous edema in the medial femoral condyle can also be seen in some cases.[22] There is a high association of concurrent lateral knee friction syndromes in the posteromedial friction syndrome patient population with a reported 25% of patients having both entities.[22] Treatment is typically conservative and symptoms respond well to corticosteroid or anesthetic injection.[36]

Popliteal tendon impingement

Popliteal tendon impingent is an uncommon disease process that is seen in patients with concurrent abnormality of the lateral femoral condyle, such as prominent osteophytes or in patients who have undergone total knee arthroplasty. These patients present with lateral knee pain, focal tenderness with palpation during knee flexion/

extension, and mechanical snapping of the tendon with activity. Pain is exacerbated by movements where the tendon passes over the osteophyte or other protruding structure resulting in chronic inflammation and injury to the tendon.[37,38] MR imaging findings suggestive of popliteal tendon impingement include abnormal signal or morphology of the popliteus tendon with adjacent protruding abnormality of the lateral femoral condyle. Because of the dynamic nature of this disease process, ultrasound may be the most useful imaging modality in making a diagnosis of popliteal tendon impingement and observing tendon snapping.[39]

SUMMARY

Several soft tissue structures about the knee may be impinged on because of the complex joint motion and number of structures in a confined space (**Table 2**). MR imaging is a frequently used tool in evaluating a patient with knee pain. Although osteoarthritis, ligamentous, or meniscal pathology are the most frequently encountered disease processes in knee MR imaging, it is paramount for the radiologist to distinguish potential surgically managed entities from other potential nonsurgical causes of knee pain including plical pathology and impingement syndromes.

CLINICS CARE POINTS

- Synovial plicae are normal structures commonly identified at MR imaging and at arthroscopy. Acute trauma and chronic repetitive injury can cause painful irritation of synovial plicae known as plica syndrome; this is most commonly seen with the medial patellar plica.

- Edema and enlargement of the suprapatellar fat pad is seen in asymptomatic populations and imaging findings should be correlated with clinical signs and symptoms of fat pad impingement.
- A pitfall in diagnosing ITB friction syndrome is misidentification of normal joint fluid within the lateral synovial recess as pathologic fluid. Fluid secondary to ITB friction syndrome should be located immediately lateral or posterior to the lateral femoral epicondyle.

DISCLOSURE

The authors have no conflicts of interest to disclose.

REFERENCES

1. Ogata S, Uhthoff HK. The development of synovial plicae in human knee joints: an embryologic study. Arthroscopy 1990;6(4):315–21.
2. Geraghty RM, Spear M. Evidence for plical support of the patella. J Anat 2017;231(5):698–707.
3. Norris M, Corbo G, Banga K, et al. The biomechanical and morphological characteristics of the ligamentum mucosum and its potential role in anterior knee pain. Knee 2018;25(6):1134–41.
4. Boles CA, Martin DF. Synovial plicae in the knee. AJR Am J Roentgenol 2001;177(1):221–7.
5. Schindler OS. The sneaky plica' revisited: morphology, pathophysiology and treatment of synovial plicae of the knee. Knee Surg Sports Traumatol Arthrosc 2014;22(2):247–62.
6. Kim SJ, Min BH, Kim HK. Arthroscopic anatomy of the infrapatellar plica. Arthroscopy 1996;12(5):561–4.
7. Patel SJ, Kaplan PA, Dussault RG, et al. Anatomy and clinical significance of the horizontal cleft in the infrapatellar fat pad of the knee: MR imaging. AJR Am J Roentgenol 1998;170(6):1551–5.
8. Kosarek FJ, Helms CA. The MR appearance of the infrapatellar plica. AJR Am J Roentgenol 1999;172(2):481–4.
9. Sakakibara JO. Arthroscopic study on Iino's band (plica synovialis mediopatellaris). J Jap Orthop Ass 1976;50:513–22.
10. Gandolfi MM R, Pegreffi P, Armaroli D. Syndrome della plica sinoiale clinica diagnosi terapia [Italian]. Chir Organi Mov 1982;68:603–13.
11. Deutsch AL, Resnick D, Dalinka MK, et al. Synovial plicae of the knee. Radiology 1981;141(3):627–34.
12. Zidorn T. Classification of the suprapatellar septum considering ontogenetic development. Arthroscopy 1992;8(4):459–64.
13. Pipkin G. Knee injuries: the role of the suprapatellar plica and suprapatellar bursa in simulating internal derangements. Clin Orthop Relat Res 1971;74:161–76.
14. Garcia-Valtuille R, Abascal F, Cerezal L, et al. Anatomy and MR imaging appearances of synovial plicae of the knee. Radiographics 2002;22(4):775–84.
15. Dupont JY. Synovial plicae of the knee. Controversies and review. Clin Sports Med 1997;16(1):87–122.
16. Cothran RL, McGuire PM, Helms CA, et al. MR imaging of infrapatellar plica injury. AJR Am J Roentgenol 2003;180(5):1443–7.
17. Griffith CJ, LaPrade RF. Medial plica irritation: diagnosis and treatment. Curr Rev Musculoskelet Med 2008;1(1):53–60.
18. Hardaker WT, Whipple TL, Bassett FH 3rd. Diagnosis and treatment of the plica syndrome of the knee. J Bone Joint Surg Am 1980;62(2):221–5.
19. Gulati A, McElrath C, Wadhwa V, et al. Current clinical, radiological and treatment perspectives of patellofemoral pain syndrome. Br J Radiol 2018;91(1086):20170456.
20. Jacobson JA, Lenchik L, Ruhoy MK, et al. MR imaging of the infrapatellar fat pad of Hoffa. Radiographics 1997;17(3):675–91.
21. Hannon J, Bardenett S, Singleton S, et al. Evaluation, treatment, and rehabilitation implications of the infrapatellar fat pad. Sports Health 2016;8(2):167–71.
22. Khan I, Ashraf T, Saifuddin A. Magnetic resonance imaging of impingement and friction syndromes around the knee. Skeletal Radiol Jun 2020;49(6):823–36.
23. Shabshin N, Schweitzer ME, Morrison WB. Quadriceps fat pad edema: significance on magnetic resonance images of the knee. Skeletal Radiol 2006;35(5):269–74.
24. Roth C, Jacobson J, Jamadar D, et al. Quadriceps fat pad signal intensity and enlargement on MRI: prevalence and associated findings. AJR Am J Roentgenol 2004;182(6):1383–7.
25. Tsavalas N, Karantanas AH. Suprapatellar fat-pad mass effect: MRI findings and correlation with anterior knee pain. AJR Am J Roentgenol 2013;200(3):W291–6.
26. Koyama S, Tensho K, Shimodaira H, et al. A case of prefemoral fat pad impingement syndrome caused by hyperplastic fat pad. Case Rep Orthop 2018;2018:3583049.
27. Ryu KN, Jaovisidha S, Schweitzer M, et al. MR imaging of lipoma arborescens of the knee joint. AJR Am J Roentgenol 1996;167(5):1229–32.
28. Soder RB, Mizerkowski MD, Petkowicz R, et al. MRI of the knee in asymptomatic adolescent swimmers: a controlled study. Br J Sports Med 2012;46(4):268–72.
29. Bohnsack M, Klages P, Hurschler C, et al. Influence of an infrapatellar fat pad edema on patellofemoral

biomechanics and knee kinematics: a possible relation to the anterior knee pain syndrome. Arch Orthop Trauma Surg 2009;129(8):1025–30.

30. Chung CB, Skaf A, Roger B, et al. Patellar tendon-lateral femoral condyle friction syndrome: MR imaging in 42 patients. Skeletal Radiol 2001;30(12):694–7.

31. Saddik D, McNally EG, Richardson M. MRI of Hoffa's fat pad. Skeletal Radiol 2004;33(8):433–44.

32. Orchard JW, Fricker PA, Abud AT, et al. Biomechanics of iliotibial band friction syndrome in runners. Am J Sports Med 1996;24(3):375–9.

33. Murphy BJ, Hechtman KS, Uribe JW, et al. Iliotibial band friction syndrome: MR imaging findings. Radiology 1992;185(2):569–71.

34. Muhle C, Ahn JM, Yeh L, et al. Iliotibial band friction syndrome: MR imaging findings in 16 patients and MR arthrographic study of six cadaveric knees. Radiology 1999;212(1):103–10.

35. Simeone FJ, Huang AJ, Chang CY, et al. Posteromedial knee friction syndrome: an entity with medial knee pain and edema between the femoral condyle, sartorius and gracilis. Skeletal Radiol 2015;44(4):557–63.

36. Simeone FJ, Kheterpal A, Chang CY, et al. Ultrasound-guided injection for the diagnosis and treatment of posteromedial knee friction syndrome. Skeletal Radiol 2019;48(4):563–8.

37. Gaine WJ, Mohammed A. Osteophyte impingement of the popliteus tendon as a cause of lateral knee joint pain. Knee 2002;9(3):249–52.

38. Shukla DR, Levy BA, Kuzma SA, et al. Snapping popliteus tendon within an osteochondritis dissecans lesion: an unusual case of lateral knee pain. Am J Orthop (Belle Mead Nj) 2014;43(9):E210–3.

39. Marchand AJ, Proisy M, Ropars M, et al. Snapping knee: imaging findings with an emphasis on dynamic sonography. AJR Am J Roentgenol 2012;199(1):142–50.

MRI of the Knee Meniscus

Lukas M. Trunz, MD, William B. Morrison, MD*

KEYWORDS

- Knee • MRI • Meniscus • Meniscus anatomy • Meniscus tear • Secondary signs • Pitfalls

KEY POINTS

- Meniscus pathology is associated with variable clinical symptoms and constitutes the most common indication among patients undergoing knee arthroscopy.
- Meniscus anatomy and composition including supporting ligaments and capsular attachments is nuanced and intricate allowing the menisci to fulfill their different functions but also resulting in diagnostic challenges.
- Radiologist will be confronted with variable appearances when imaging menisci and should therefore be familiar with anatomy, injury mechanisms and protocol considerations, and meniscal tear patterns including secondary signs/pitfalls.
- Meniscal tears can be associated with meniscal extrusion and displaced fragments, and can lead to secondary osteoarthritis or result in subchondral insufficiency fracture with possible osteonecrosis.

INTRODUCTION

The medial and lateral menisci of the knee are crescent-shaped fibrocartilaginous structures located between the femoral condyles and the tibial plateau, partially dividing the joint cavity. When interpreting knee MRIs meniscal pathology is frequently encountered, specifically meniscal tears based on degeneration or acute knee trauma. Indeed, prior research has shown that meniscal tears constitute nearly 50% of all indications among patients undergoing knee arthroscopies.[1] Dependent on the mechanism and other concurrent tibiofemoral pathology, patients with meniscal dysfunction present clinically with variable symptoms including pain, stiffness, swelling, locking, instability ("giving way" of the knee), or hearing/sensation of a "pop" during trauma which might be associated with a simultaneous anterior cruciate ligament (ACL) tear.[2,3] This article reviews meniscal anatomy, injury mechanisms, and important MRI protocol considerations. We also outline the different types of meniscal tears including secondary signs, diagnostic pitfalls, as well as current surgical treatment options.

ANATOMY
Composition and Internal Architecture

To allow the menisci to fulfill their different functions, they have a unique biochemical composition. The meniscus fibrocartilage is a dense extracellular matrix (ECM) that is mainly composed of water (72%), collagen (22%), proteoglycans, and glycoproteins.[4,5] Collagen accounts for up to 75% of the dry weight of the ECM and most of the collagen fibers represent type I collagen.[4] These fibers are organized in 3 distinct layers and are found predominantly in the deepest of the 3 layers in a circumferential orientation. This enables the menisci to provide tensile strength and resist hoop stresses, which is essential to evenly distribute weight across the joint as load-bearing occurs. Radially orientated "tie" fibers are present in the middle layer, as well as woven in between circumferential fibers in the deep layer, to supply additional structural integrity besides resistance to longitudinal splitting and shear forces. Finally, the thin surface layer is most superficial and contributes to a smooth and gliding surface.[4–7]

Department of Radiology, Thomas Jefferson University Hospital, Main Building, 132 S 10th, Street, Philadelphia, PA 19107, USA
* Corresponding author.
E-mail address: William.morrison@jefferson.edu
Twitter: @MorrisonMSK (W.B.M.)

Magn Reson Imaging Clin N Am 30 (2022) 307–324
https://doi.org/10.1016/j.mric.2021.11.009
1064-9689/22/© 2021 Elsevier Inc. All rights reserved.

Vascular Anatomy

In standard anatomy, a total of 5 genicular arteries, namely, the paired superior medial and superior lateral genicular arteries, inferior medial and inferior lateral genicular arteries as well as the single middle genicular artery, originate from the midportion of the popliteal artery and supply blood to the knee.[8] The menisci themselves are largely avascular structures; however, a perimeniscal capillary plexus penetrates the peripheral meniscal borders and thereby vascularizes the peripheral 10% to 30% of the menisci, also known as "red zone."[6,9] This distinct vascular anatomy plays a crucial part in meniscal healing with tears located in the central avascular zones being less likely to undergo healing. The central inner portion of the menisci, also known as the "white zone," receives nourishment mainly via synovial diffusion which is facilitated by joint movement.[4,6] It should be noted that the vascular anatomy in children differs from adults. The fetal meniscus is entirely vascularized at birth; however, the vascularity subsequently gradually decreases, and by the age of 10 to 12 years essentially resembles the adult meniscus.[7,10]

Configuration and Attachments

Each meniscus consists of an anterior horn, body, and posterior horn, and is anchored to the tibial plateau at their anterior/posterior root attachments.

The larger, medial meniscus (MM) measures approximately between 40 and 45 mm in length, 27 mm in width, and covers 51% to 74% of the medial articular surface. The MM has a more open C-shape configuration with the posterior horn being larger than the anterior horn (**Fig. 1**). In comparison, the lateral meniscus (LM) anterior and posterior horns are similar in size/shape in cross-section. Further, the LM is almost circular and measures between 32 and 35 mm in length, noting that the LM, however, covers a larger area of the lateral tibial articular surface at 75% to 93%.[5,6]

The posterior horn of the MM is tightly attached to the posterior intercondylar area of the tibia just anterior to the insertion of the posterior cruciate ligament (PCL), while the anterior horn has a more variable insertion anterior to the ACL. For the LM, the attachment of the anterior horn is adjacent and lateral to the ACL, and the posterior horn attachment is adjacent and slightly anterior to that of the posterior horn of the MM.[11] The roots of the menisci are ligament-like structures that anchor the meniscal horns to the tibial plateau. They prevent meniscal extrusion (outward displacement)

and provide secondary stability, and therefore are critical in maintaining the biomechanical properties of the knee joint.[12,13]

Supporting Ligaments and Capsular Attachments

Meniscofemoral ligaments

The meniscofemoral ligaments (MFL) connect the posterior horn of the LM with the intercondylar portion of the medial femoral condyle. These ligaments consist of the anterior (Humphrey) and posterior (Wrisberg) ligaments, which run anterior and posterior to the PCL, respectively. The presence of the MFLs is highly variable; a prior systematic literature review by Gupte and colleagues showed that of 1022 cadaveric knees, 91% had at least one MFL, and hence the presence of at least one MFL should be considered normal. Both ligaments coexisted in approximately 32%.[14] Besides their inconsistent presence, there remains uncertainty about the function of these ligaments; it has been proposed that they protect and stabilize the posterior horn, preventing the excess displacement of the LM in various settings.[14,15] On MRI, the insertion of the MFL to the posterior horn of the LM can create the appearance of a "pseudo-tear," which must be differentiated from a true tear in this location that occurs typically in the setting of an ACL injury and is referred to as "Wrisberg rip."[16]

Medial Collateral Ligament and Capsular Structures

The medial collateral ligament (MCL) extends from the medial epicondyle of the femur to the medial condyle of the tibia. In contrast to the lateral collateral ligament, the MCL is fixed to the MM as well as the joint capsule. Therefore, the MM is less mobile, not surrounded by fluid peripherally, and much more injury-prone compared with the LM. The attachments of the MCL and MM compose the deep portions of the MCL and consist of 2 parts; the MFL (coronary ligament), and the meniscotibial ligament.[17]

Laterally, fibrous bands (meniscal-popliteal fascicles) originate from the popliteus tendon sheath and connect to the posterior horn of the LM. They contribute to forming the popliteal hiatus and limit excessive forward motion of the LM during knee extension.[18]

MECHANICS AND MECHANISM OF INJURY

The menisci play a crucial role to compensate for the physiologic incongruence of the femoral and tibial articular surfaces and help distribute axial

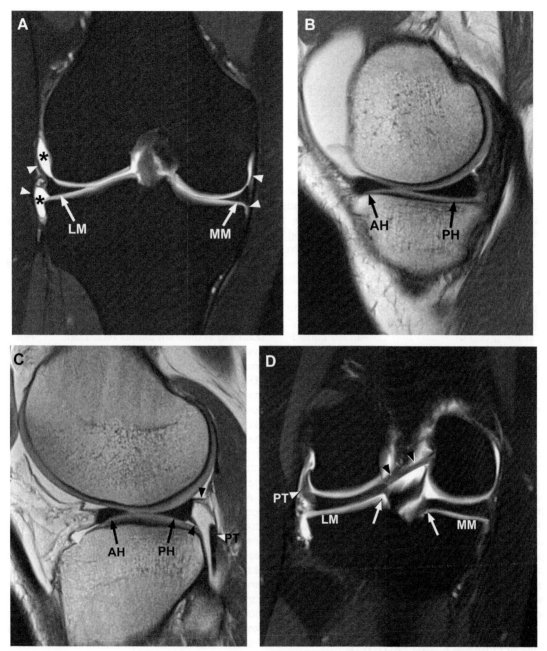

Fig. 1. Meniscal anatomy. (*A*) Coronal fat-suppressed T1-weighted MR arthrographic image through the middle of the joint shows normal meniscal anatomy. (MM = medial meniscus; LM = lateral meniscus; *arrowheads* = meniscocapsular attachments; *asterisks* = perimeniscal joint recesses). Note that the capsular attachments are looser laterally with larger, more distensible joint recesses. (*B*) Sagittal proton density MR image through the medial compartment shows the normal triangular configuration of the medial meniscus. The posterior horn of the medial meniscus (PH) is larger than the anterior horn (AH). (*C*) Sagittal proton density MR image through the lateral compartment shows the normal triangular configuration of the lateral meniscus. The posterior horn (PH) is similar size as the anterior horn (AH). Note the popliteal-meniscal fascicles (*arrowheads*) and the adjacent popliteus tendon (PT). (*D*) Coronal fat-suppressed T1-weighted MR arthrographic image through the posterior aspect of the joint shows normal meniscal root attachments (*arrows*). Note posterior meniscofemoral ligament (Wrisberg, black *arrowheads*) extending from the posterior horn of the lateral meniscus to the medial femoral condyle, and the popliteus tendon (PT) coursing through the popliteal hiatus next to the lateral meniscus. (MM = medial meniscus; LM = lateral meniscus).

loading across the knee joint. In addition, they protect the articular surfaces from mechanical damage by shock absorption and contribute to secondary joint stabilization, lubrication, and nutrient distribution.[4,6,12,19]

Different mechanisms of injuries to the knee have different effects on the menisci. The commonly seen pivot-shift injury refers to the anterior tibial translation relative to the femur, which is often associated with the disruption of the ACL. It has been theorized that in this scenario simultaneous contraction of the semimembranosus muscle creates opposing forces on the MM most commonly leading to the peripheral tearing of the MM near the meniscocapsular attachment. Moreover, if enough valgus displacement occurs during ACL injury, the LM posterior horn and body are squeezed between the femur and tibia, which may result in LM tears.[20,21] While various tear patterns are observed in ACL injuries, peripheral vertical MM tears at the posterior horn represent the most commonly encountered tear morphology, and the group of Vinson and colleagues considered the presence of peripheral vertical meniscal tears as a highly specific secondary sign for an acute or chronic ACL injury.[22]

In addition, prior studies have also shown a frequent association of meniscal injuries with femoral shaft fractures as well as tibial plateau fractures. MR imaging can be useful in assessing the full extent of injury regarding meniscal tear, displacement, and entrapment, especially in patients whereby the clinical examination is limited.[23,24] Meniscal entrapment has also been described in the context of tibial spine avulsion fractures.[25] While these fractures are uncommon in the adult population, the radiologist should have a high index of suspicion for meniscal entrapment in pediatric patients, particularly in partially displaced or hinged (type II) and completely displaced (type III) tibial spine avulsion fractures, as prior research has suggested a low detection rate on MRI.[26]

MRI APPEARANCE AND PROTOCOL CONSIDERATIONS

MRI provides excellent soft-tissue contrast and, therefore, is the test of choice for evaluating internal knee derangements including meniscal pathology noninvasively. On both coronal and sagittal images, the anterior/posterior horns of the menisci resemble low signal intensity triangles, and, on sagittal imaging, demonstrate the classic "bowtie" appearance in the periphery. In the absence of prior debridement, the posterior horn of the MM is larger than the anterior horn, noting that the horns of the LM are similar in size and shape.

Protocol considerations for the detection of meniscal pathology should optimally include the use of high field (greater than 1.0 T) MRI and dedicated surface coils. To achieve high-spatial resolution, the typical parameters include a field of view of 14 to 16 cm, a matrix size of at least 256 x 256, and a slice thickness of 3 to 4 mm. For the accurate detection of meniscal tears, both proton-density as well as T2-weighted sequences are vital and complementary. Further, three-dimensional (3D) sequences with near-isotropic resolution have recently gained more attention in the musculoskeletal radiology literature. While two-dimensional (2D) fast spin-echo (FSE) sequences provide high in-plane spatial resolution and superb tissue contrast, partial volume averaging remains a challenge compared with 3D sequences with thinner slices and associated reduced partial volume averaging effects. Furthermore, with 3D imaging, multiplanar reformations in a variety of planes can be created from the source data after a single acquisition, making repeat scanning in different planes redundant.[19,27] However, despite these advantages, a recent meta-analysis by Shakoor and colleagues showed that 3D sequences have a similar diagnostic performance compared with currently used 2D sequences.[28] To evaluate for recurrent meniscal tears in the postoperative setting after partial meniscectomy/meniscus repair, MR arthrography is preferred over conventional MRI for patients with meniscal resection involving 25% or more of the meniscus.[29]

As with other body parts imaged, MRI artifacts occur and limit the diagnostic potential of the study. Motion artifact is seen daily in a busy practice and can be counteracted by decreasing imaging time or providing more effective immobilization of the limb. Vascular motion from the popliteal artery can be minimized by applying a saturation band above the field of view. Additionally, several motion compensation techniques have been developed, such as oversampling the center of k-space (eg, blade or propeller) that provides redundant information for error correction, and, subsequently, sequences contributing to motion can be identified and removed.[30] Another artifact occasionally encountered is blur artifact in low TE FSE sequences if a high echo train length is also used. This could potentially lead to missed subtle/linear findings (eg, meniscal tears). An increased TE (over 25 ms) and lower echo train length (eg, 4) can eliminate this artifact.

CT arthrography plays an essential role in the evaluation of meniscal tears in patients with a contraindication to MRI (eg, pacemaker, claustrophobia, presence of metal in the area of interest) and is an acceptable alternative if an MRI cannot be completed.[31] Ultrasound (US) of the knee for the assessment of meniscal pathologies is not routinely used; however, US can be useful to detect meniscal extrusion and parameniscal cysts.[32]

Discoid Meniscus

One variation of meniscal morphology is of clinical importance: the *discoid* meniscus.[33,34] Nearly 100% of the time this involves the LM (**Fig. 2**). The incidence is difficult to estimate as clinical imaging represents a biased population but more importantly, there are many different criteria used for diagnosis. Reported incidence of 0.3% to 17% is as wide as it is obviously flawed. "Less than 1%" is a good rule of thumb. A discoid meniscus has a spectrum of configurations leading to confusion. The classic discoid meniscus is "pancake" shaped, extending across the lateral compartment toward the tibial spine with uniform thickness. This variant is highly susceptible to tear early in life. At the other end of the spectrum is a meniscus that is relatively normal in configuration but one which extends more central than normal. Measurements have been proposed including meniscal body width of 15 mm or more on a midline coronal image or a ratio of the meniscal width to the tibial width of more than 20%. The borderline cases that represent a measurement challenge are likely not any more susceptible to tear than one with normal measurements.

Meniscal Ossicle

A meniscal ossicle was once thought to represent another variation; it is not really an ossicle, although it may resemble one or an intra-articular body on radiographs. This entity actually represents the ossification of a portion of the meniscal substance, most commonly involving the posterior horn of the MM (**Fig. 3**). Historically this was thought to represent a normal variation of meniscal development, but it was a mystery why they were not seen in the pediatric population. The mystery was solved shortly after meniscal root tears were described, along with cases in which ossification seemed on follow-up examinations after a root tear was diagnosed. Meniscal ossicle is now considered to be dystrophic ossification (or healing response) of a torn meniscal segment, usually following a large tear of the root attachment.[35]

MENISCAL TEAR
Diagnostic Criteria

MRI has proven to be a highly accurate diagnostic tool for the detection of meniscal tears. To diagnose a meniscal tear one of the 2 criteria have to be fulfilled: Intrasubstance signal alteration extending to the superior or inferior articular surface, or abnormal meniscal morphology. If these findings are present on at least 2 consecutive slices (either 2 sagittal, 2 coronals, or on one sagittal and one coronal) meniscal tears can be diagnosed with greater than 90% accuracy and should be reported as such.[36]

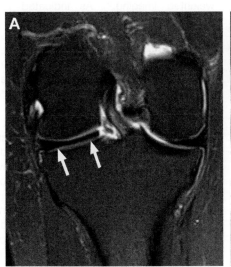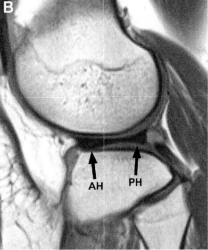

Fig. 2. Discoid meniscus. (*A*) Coronal fat-suppressed proton density MR image shows the extension of lateral meniscal substance (*arrows*) nearly to the intercondylar notch, representing a discoid meniscus.(*B*) Sagittal proton density MR image through the midportion of lateral compartment shows the confluence of the anterior horn (AH) and posterior horn (PH) representing discoid configuration.

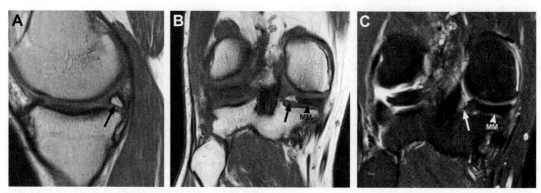

Fig. 3. Meniscal ossicle. (*A*) Sagittal proton density MR image through the medial compartment shows the ossification of the posterior horn of the medial meniscus (*arrow*). (*B*). Coronal T1-weighted MR image shows ossification (*arrow*) of the medial meniscus (MM) near the posterior root attachment. (*C*) Coronal fat-suppressed proton density MR image shows posterior root tear (*arrow*) of the medial meniscus (MM) associated with meniscal ossicle formation.

However, if findings are only seen on one slice, accuracy decreases markedly, and a possible tear should be reported. The differential diagnosis for signal alteration not extending to the articular surface includes myxoid degeneration, normal vascularity (predominantly in children/young adults), and acute contusion after trauma.[19] Similar to other areas in radiology, artificial intelligence has made its impact on clinically orientated musculoskeletal radiological tasks. For the diagnosis of meniscal tears, Fritz and colleagues showed that deep convolutional neural networks have a similar specificity, but a lower sensitivity compared with fellowship-trained musculoskeletal radiologists for the detection of surgically proven meniscus tears.[37] Morphology of tear has treatment and prognostic implications and should be included in the report. Tear types and subtypes are discussed later in discussion and summarized in **Fig. 4**.

Longitudinal Tears

Longitudinally oriented meniscal tears include horizontal, oblique, and vertical tears; thus, to prevent ambiguity, it is important to describe the specific tear morphology when discussing longitudinal meniscal tears.

Vertical Longitudinal Tears

Vertical longitudinal tears (VLTs) follow the long axis of the meniscus in a perpendicular orientation to the tibial plateau, hence dividing the meniscus into central and peripheral portions[19] (**Fig. 5**). Often seen in younger/active individuals in the setting of a knee injury, they can involve one or both articular surfaces and present on MRI as linear vertically orientated increased intrameniscal signal. These tears are most commonly located in

the posterior horn of the MM and involve the peripheral third of the meniscus. When associated with ACL tear and pivot-shift mechanism, this tear is referred to as a "ramp lesion." VLTs may extend into the body and anterior horn of the meniscus, which increases the risk for a meniscal fragment to displace or flip, for example, a bucket-handle tear.[38,39] Peripheral VLTs (PVLTs) near the meniscocapsular junction have an increased capability for spontaneous healing related to the presence of vascularity in that location, and the group of Kijowski and colleagues has shown that MRI can be used to assess the healing potential of PVLTs using MRI characteristics such as the width of the tear (<2 mm) or the presence of low-signal strands bridging the tear on T2-weighted imaging.[40] As indicated previously, PVLTs have a high association with ACL injuries referred to as "ramp lesions." Definitions of ramp lesions vary, however, in a recent work by Greif and colleagues, ramp lesions were defined as a longitudinal tear pattern within the posterior horn of the MM and/or the meniscocapsular/meniscotibial ligaments.[41] Multiple factors such as knee extension during imaging and different imaging appearances contribute to the low sensitivity for the detection of ramp lesions on MRI, and arthroscopy represents the gold standard. However, evaluating ramp lesions during arthroscopy also comes with challenges.[42] Because ramp lesions are associated with biomechanical instability, these tears may predispose to ACL graft failure and further articular damage, and radiologists need to be familiar with this specific type of tear.[41]

Horizontal Tears

Horizontal tears (HTs), also called horizontal cleavage tears, extend usually from the free edge of the

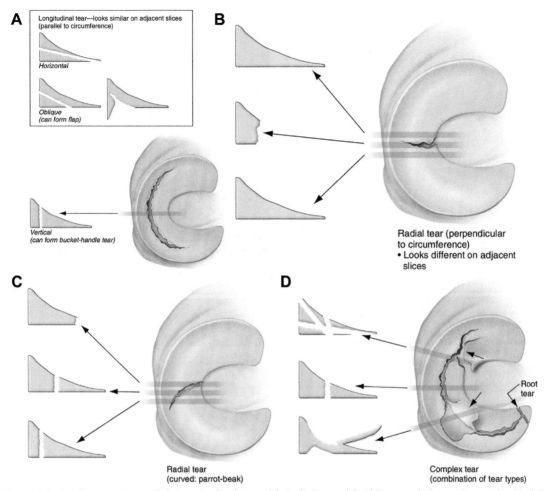

Fig. 4. Meniscal tear patterns. (*A*) Longitudinal tear. (*B*) Radial tear. (*C*) Oblique radial tear (parrot-beak). (*D*) Complex tear. (Please use Elsevier Problem Solving in Musculoskeletal Imaging, Morrison WB and Sanders TG, Figure 12–35).

meniscus to the periphery and are parallel orientated to the tibial plateau, thus dissecting the meniscus into superior and inferior portions (**Fig. 6**). They are more commonly seen in individuals older than 40 years on a degenerative basis without an associated discrete knee injury. On MRI they seem as abnormal horizontal linear signal that contacts the meniscal surface or free edge. HTs are often better seen on short TE sequences; however, surface extension might be subtle and signal intensity of fluid on T2-weighted sequences increases diagnostic certainty. The presence of a parameniscal cyst often indicates the presence of at least a HT component that extends to the periphery and allows direct communication with joint fluid.[19,38,39,43]

Oblique longitudinal tears are a subset of HTs that typically extend to the undersurface (tibial articular surface) of the meniscus instead of the free edge. These tears are very common at the posterior horn and body of the MM. Configuration of this tear can lead to characteristic displaced flap fragments extending from the meniscal body into the adjacent meniscotibial recess (often called the "boomerang sign" or "meniscal comma sign") and from the posterior horn into the intercondylar notch (**Fig. 7**).

Radial Tears

Radial tears are perpendicularly orientated to both the tibial plateau and the long axis of the meniscus and arise from the free edge of the meniscus (**Fig. 8**). They occur in the avascular "white zone" and have therefore a low likelihood to undergo healing and are therefore repaired less frequently. An important differentiating feature compared with longitudinal tears is, that radial tears disrupt the circumferential collagen fibers and subsequent loss of hoop strength results often in meniscal extrusion.[44] Dependent on the scan plane and location of the tear several imaging patterns can

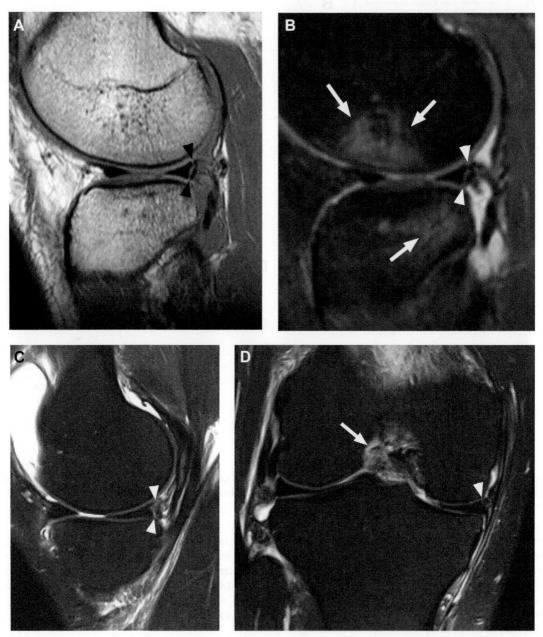

Fig. 5. Vertical longitudinal tear. (*A., B*). Sagittal proton density (*A*) and sagittal fat-suppressed proton density (*B*) MR images through the lateral compartment in a patient with ACL tear show a vertical, peripheral tear (*arrowheads*) of the lateral meniscus. Note characteristic bone bruise pattern (*arrows*) associated with pivot-shift mechanism of injury. (*C., D*). Sagittal fat-suppressed proton density MR image through the medial compartment (*C*) and coronal fat-suppressed proton density MR image through the midjoint (*D*) of a different patient than figure a and b show a vertical, peripheral tear (*arrowheads*) of the posterior horn and body of the medial meniscus (the "ramp lesion"). Note ACL tear on the coronal image (*arrow*).

be observed with radial tears on MRI including a "cleft" or "truncated meniscus" sign. Also, often as a result of a full-thickness radial tear, a "ghost meniscus" sign can be seen on sagittal or coronal images, with the apparent absence of the meniscus on one slice between 2 normal-appearing slices.[19,44] Axial sequences can be very helpful as well in assessing radial tears and estimating their depth. Oblique radial tears, referred to as "parrot beak" tears, are described when radial tears curve into a longitudinal orientation[43] (**Fig. 9**). This can cause an inwardly

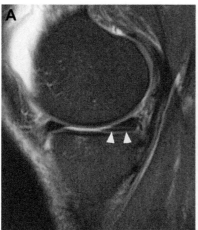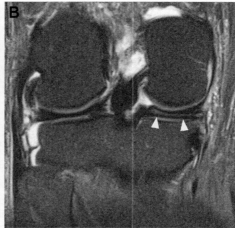

Fig. 6. Horizontal tear. (*A., B*). Sagittal (*A*) and coronal (*B*) fat-suppressed proton density MR images show linear signal extending transversely through the posterior horn of the medial meniscus, separating the meniscus into upper and lower portions, representing a horizontal tear.

displaced free-edge flap, similar in appearance to a parrot's beak.[45] It should be noted, however, that this appearance is better appreciated on arthroscopy and some authors advocate not to use the term "parrot beak" in the MR description of a meniscal tear pattern.[38]

Root Tears

Meniscal root tears have gained more attention in the orthopedic/musculoskeletal radiology world over the last decade as studies have shown that root tears cause significantly increased contact pressure across the joint and have a higher association with sequelae such as subchondral insufficiency fractures.[44,46] Radial tears constitute the vast majority of root tears, which most commonly occur at the posterior horn of the MM and LM (**Fig. 10**). While more commonly observed in the MM on a degenerative basis, posterior root tears involving the LM are often associated with ACL injuries.[39,47] On MRI both sagittal and coronal sequences are crucial for the accurate assessment

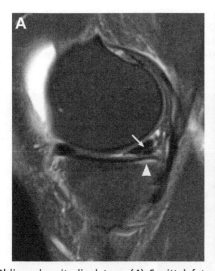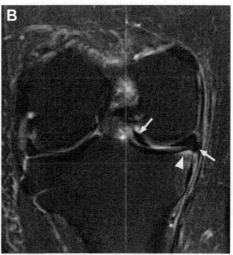

Fig. 7. Oblique longitudinal tear. (*A*) Sagittal fat-suppressed proton density MR image through the medial compartment shows linear signal (*arrow*) extending obliquely through the posterior horn of the medial meniscus to the inferior border representing an oblique, longitudinal tear. (*B*) Coronal fat-suppressed proton density MR image of the same patient shows displaced flap fragments (*arrows*) in the meniscotibial recess ("boomerang sign" or "meniscal comma sign") and in the intercondylar notch. This displaced flap pattern is common in cases of oblique longitudinal tear of the medial meniscus. Note linear, subchondral bone marrow edema (*arrowheads* in a. and b.) in the tibial plateau adjacent to the meniscus, a useful secondary sign of a meniscal tear.

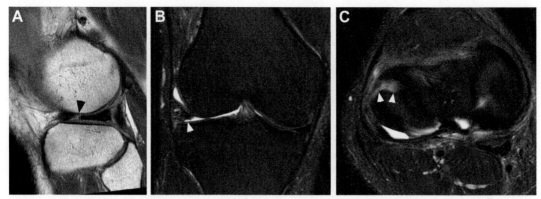

Fig. 8. Radial tear. (*A*) Sagittal proton density MR image through the lateral compartment shows vertical, linear signal (*arrowhead*) through the body of the lateral meniscus representing a radial tear. (*B*) Coronal fat-suppressed proton density MR image of the same patient through the radial tear shows the truncation of lateral meniscal substance (*arrowhead*). (*C*) Axial fat-suppressed proton density MR image depicts the tear (*arrowheads*) in the transverse imaging plane.

of root tears: A vertical fluid cleft on coronal imaging and the "ghost meniscus" sign on sagittal imaging are commonly identified.[38] Although not specific, many complete root tears are unstable and result in a major loss of hoop strength, with significant meniscal extrusion (extension of the meniscal body > 3 mm beyond the edge of the tibial plateau on a midcoronal MRI),[43] which can, in turn, lead to rapidly progressive articular cartilage damage or subchondral stress fracture.

Complex Tears

Complex tears exhibit more than one tear plane previously discussed (**Fig. 11**). Although these can be referred to on the report as complex tears, an attempt should be made to add a description of

the predominant tear plane, especially one associated with flap formation or instability (ie, radial tear or root tear) to help the orthopedic surgeon with preoperative treatment planning. Kise and colleagues showed that complex tears are associated with worse outcomes after 1 and 2 years postpartial meniscectomy than other tears.[48]

Displaced Tears

Although the radiologist must evaluate every knee MRI for displaced meniscal tears, this becomes especially important when a diminutive meniscus is encountered in the absence of prior meniscal surgery. Clinically displaced meniscal tears can present with persistent knee pain and locking, often requiring surgical treatment. The spectrum

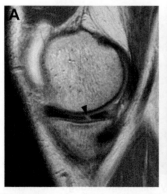
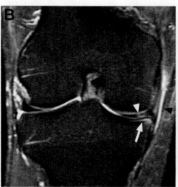
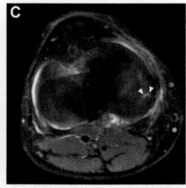

Fig. 9. Parrot-beak tear. (*A*) Sagittal proton density MR image through the medial compartment shows vertical, linear signal (*arrowhead*) through the body of the medial meniscus. (*B*) Coronal fat-suppressed proton density MR image of the same patient also shows linear signal (white *arrowhead*) through the medial meniscus as the radial tear curves along the medial meniscal substance. Note secondary signs of meniscal tear: subchondral bone marrow signal (*arrow*) and perimeniscal edema (*black arrow*). (*C*) Axial fat-suppressed proton density MR image depicts the tear (*arrowheads*) in the transverse imaging plane. Note curved configuration.

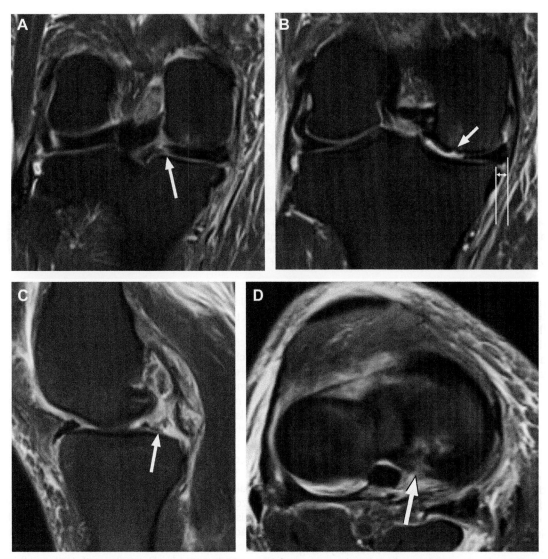

Fig. 10. Meniscal root tear and extrusion. (*A*) Coronal fat-suppressed proton density MR image shows linear signal (*arrow*) in the medial meniscus representing a radial tear through the posterior root attachment. (*B*) Coronal fat-suppressed proton density MR image of the same knee through the midjoint shows outward displacement (extrusion) of the medial meniscal body (*lines, double-headed arrow*) from the margin of the tibial plateau. Note chondrosis and subchondral bone marrow edema, which in addition to meniscal extrusion represent sequelae and secondary signs of meniscal tear. c., d. Sagittal (*C*) and axial (*D*) fat-suppressed proton density MR images through the tear show the disruption of meniscal signal (*arrows*) at the posterior root attachment.

of displaced tears includes free fragments, displaced flap tears, and bucket-handle tears.[19] Location and origin of the flap fragment should be described in the report. A common flap fragment has been described above, related to an oblique longitudinal tear which commonly results in flaps displaced into the meniscotibial recess (the "boomerang sign") and posterior intercondylar notch (see **Fig. 7**). Large radial tears of the posterior root attachment can lead to the entire posterior horn of the MM or LM flipping into the anterior joint

recess above the anterior horn. Bucket handle tears deserve special consideration because they are common and easily overlooked (**Fig. 12**). These lesions result from VLTs or ramp lesions and are often associated with ACL tear. Occasionally a patient will present with locking months or years after ACL reconstruction, due to a bucket-handle tear resulting from an unrecognized ramp lesion that was missed on the MRI after injury. The tear can progress like a crack in a car windshield across the periphery of the meniscus,

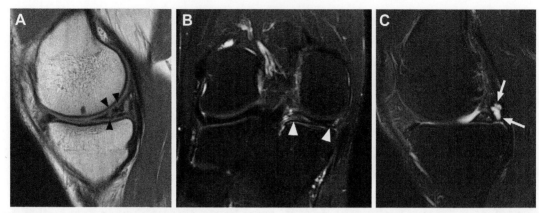

Fig. 11. Complex tear. (*A., B*). Sagittal proton density (*A*) and coronal fat-suppressed proton density (*B*) MR images show multiple tear components (*arrowheads*) through the posterior horn of the medial meniscus, representing a complex tear. (*C*) Sagittal fat-suppressed proton density MR image through the posterior horn shows a lobulated parameniscal cyst (*arrows*), a secondary sign of meniscal tear.

presenting in a delayed fashion. Bucket-handle tears are most commonly (about 95%) medial, the fragment displaced centrally into the intercondylar notch inferior to the PCL seen on sagittal images as a "double PCL sign."[49] The relatively rare lateral bucket-handle tear does not form the double PCL sign due to greater distance and intervening presence of the ACL.

Meniscal Tear: Secondary Signs

Secondary signs of meniscal tear on MRI can help diagnostically, especially when primary criteria are borderline (ie, signal extending to the surface on only one slice) or in situations when there is artifact limiting the visualization of a tear.[50] Secondary signs are based on mechanical or physiologic changes associated with the tear.

Meniscal extrusion
Meniscal extrusion (see **Fig. 10**B) was already discussed, resulting from the disruption of the circumferential fibers that provide hoop strength. Most commonly extrusion is related to radial tears, complex tears, or tears at the root attachment.[51] Measurement of extrusion greater than 3 mm ("major" extrusion) is significantly associated with tear. Minor (less than 3 mm) extrusion can occur physiologically or can be related to meniscal degeneration. In more severe cases of chronic meniscal degeneration, extrusion can exceed 3 mm.

Cartilage damage
Chondrosis in the same compartment as a questionable meniscal tear is associated with meniscal tear; this sign is especially specific when the

cartilage defect, fissure, or thinning is directly next to the meniscus (see **Fig. 10**B).

Subchondral bone marrow edema
Subchondral bone marrow edema (BME) can have different appearances related to the origin of the edema. Three types are particularly associated with meniscal tear. The first is related to overlying cartilage damage, ranging from "flame shaped" subchondral edema to cystic changes[52] (see **Fig. 10**B). This reinforces the importance of adjacent chondrosis as a secondary sign of meniscal tear. The second form of BME is less etiologically certain as to etiology. This consists of a thin, linear horizontal strip of high T2 signal directly under the meniscus, typically at the periphery of the tibial surface (see **Figs. 7**A, B, and **9**B). It may represent altered mechanics related to adjacent meniscal tear, or hyperemia. Regardless of etiology, this sign has a very high association with meniscal tear. A similar, curvilinear pattern of edema is seen with early, subtle tears of the meniscal root attachment.[53] A third type is BME due to a frank subchondral stress (insufficiency) fracture (the entity previously referred to as SONK, spontaneous osteonecrosis of the knee); this is most commonly associated with a large radial tear at the posterior root attachment with extrusion, causing the concentration of weight-bearing force at the central aspect of the tibiofemoral compartment.[54]

Parameniscal cyst
Likely the most specific secondary sign of a meniscal tear is the presence of a parameniscal cyst (see **Fig. 11**C). If detected, this sign is virtually diagnostic of underlying meniscal tear. Care must be taken to differentiate a true cyst from normal structures such as geniculate vessels and joint

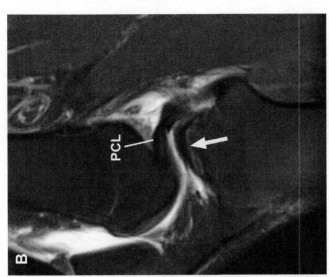

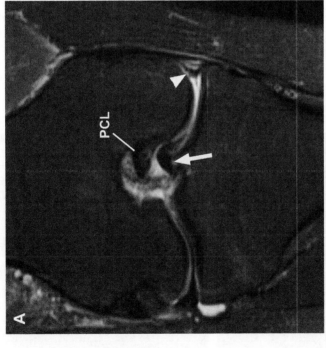

Fig. 12. Bucket-handle tear. (A) Coronal fat-suppressed proton density MR image shows truncation (*arrowhead*) of the medial meniscus with a bucket-handle fragment (*arrow*) displaced into the intercondylar notch. (PCL = posterior cruciate ligament). (*B*) Sagittal fat-suppressed proton density MR image through the intercondylar notch shows the displaced bucket-handle fragment (*arrow*) under the posterior cruciate ligament (PCL), resulting in the "double rainbow sign."

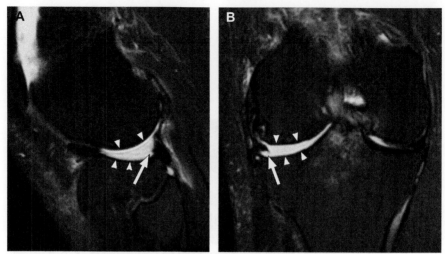

Fig. 13. Expected postoperative appearance following partial meniscectomy. (*A., B*). Sagittal (*A*) and coronal (*B*) fat-suppressed proton density MR images show the truncation of the lateral meniscus (*arrows*) along the body and posterior horn representing partial meniscectomy without recurrent tear. Note diffuse cartilage thinning (*arrowheads*) throughout the lateral compartment.

recesses. A parameniscal cyst (or meniscal cyst) demonstrates focal, rounded, or lobulated fluid signal centered at (and connected with) the periphery of the meniscus. In contrast, a joint recess is above or below the meniscal margin and generally proportionate to joint fluid. Although parameniscal cysts are highly specific for tear, they are only seen in approximately 7% of meniscal tears so sensitivity is low.[55]

Meniscal Tear: Pitfalls

Chondrocalcinosis

Chondrocalcinosis refers to the deposition of various types of crystals in cartilage, with the most common crystals representing calcium pyrophosphate dihydrate (CPPD).[56] Usually detected incidentally on radiographs typical locations for chondrocalcinosis include the menisci of the knee. While findings on MRI are often subtle, for

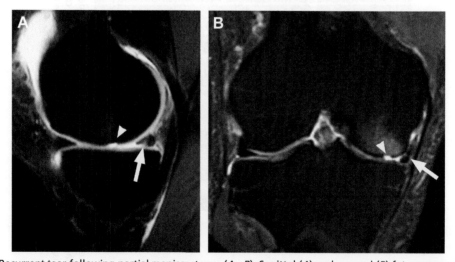

Fig. 14. Recurrent tear following partial meniscectomy. (*A., B*). Sagittal (*A*) and coronal (*B*) fat-suppressed proton density MR images show a diminutive medial meniscal body and posterior horn (*arrows*) with irregular margins and internal T2 hyperintensity representing a recurrent meniscal tear (surgically proven). Note focal cartilage defect (*arrowheads*) at the weight-bearing aspect of the medial femoral condyle with surrounding bone marrow edema.

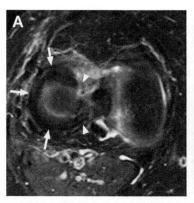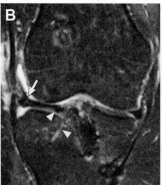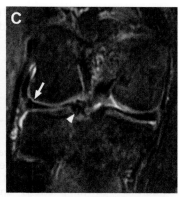

Fig. 15. Meniscal transplant. (*A–C*). Axial (*A*) and coronal (*B, C*) fat-suppressed proton density MR images show expected appearance of a transplanted lateral meniscus (*arrows*) with sutures at the root attachments (*arrowheads*).

example, due to volume averaging, chondrocalcinosis most commonly presents as discrete regions of low signal within the articular cartilage/menisci.[56,57] Furthermore, when evaluating for meniscal tears, Kaushik and colleagues suggested in their work correlation with radiographs as the presence of chondrocalcinosis has shown to decrease diagnostic accuracy on MRI.[58]

Meniscal flounce

A meniscal flounce is a well-known positional variant that usually affects the MM with an incidence of 0.2% to 0.5% on knee MRI examinations, describes a single symmetric fold along the free edge of the meniscus, and does not indicate a meniscal tear.[16,19,59] The "flounce" sign is seen significantly more often during arthroscopy because of knee positioning and is a high indicator for an intact meniscus.[19,60]

Root attachments

The meniscal root attachments can have a striated appearance and therefore might be confused with meniscal tears. Due to its proximity to the insertion of the ACL, it is especially important to be aware of this when evaluating the anterior horn of the LM to not confuse contributing ACL insertional fibers with an LM anterior horn tear.[61]

Sequelae of Meniscal Tear

As noted above, a meniscal tear with extrusion can result in subchondral insufficiency fracture. This can progress to necrosis and collapse of the articular surface.[62] Subchondral insufficiency fracture is a more likely outcome if the patient has underlying osteoporosis. If bone mineralization is normal, meniscal tear can lead to cartilage wear and secondary osteoarthritis instead, due to microinstability.

Postoperative Appearance

If the meniscal tear is unstable, surgery is usually indicated. The unstable component of tear is debrided, referred to as "partial meniscectomy." Complete meniscectomy has been abandoned due to the high incidence of secondary arthritis and subchondral fracture, a distant memory of a bygone age when the menisci were considered to be unnecessary remnants of joint development. Peripheral tears can be repaired by suturing through to the capsule using an arthroscopic approach (referred to as "all inside," "inside-out," or "outside-in" depending on method). More recently biologics and scaffold matrix materials have been incorporated to augment healing and functional restoration.[63] The postoperative meniscus should be smooth, often with truncation or blunting[64] (**Fig. 13**). Recurrent tear can be diagnosed on MRI if there is the irregularity of the surface, a meniscal flap fragment, or fluid signal within the meniscal substance (**Fig. 14**). MR arthrography can be useful to detect recurrent tear. CT arthrography is an effective modality if the patient has a contraindication to MRI.

Meniscal transplant has been attempted by a number of vendors and researchers over the past decade but is generally considered to be a procedure of last resort.[65] Meniscal transplant is seen on MRI as an otherwise relatively normal-appearing meniscus (if not retorn) with sutures or bone graft at the root attachments and surrounding capsule (**Fig. 15**). The transplant most commonly fails at the root attachment.

SUMMARY

It can be challenging to diagnose meniscal tears. Knowledge of anatomy, mechanics, and mechanisms of injury can help the Radiologist recognize pathologic patterns and sequelae of injury.

CLINICS CARE POINTS

- When encountering an ACL tear, assess for peripheral vertical medical meniscus tears involving the posterior horn which are referred to as "ramp lesions" and associated with biomechanical instability.

- Be aware that the insertion of the MFL to the posterior horn of the LM can create the appearance of a "pseudotear" which must be differentiated from a true tear often in the setting of an ACL injury ("Wrisberg rip")

- When encountering a diminutive meniscus in the absence of prior meniscal surgery, look closely for a displaced meniscal tear.

- When primary criteria for a meniscus tear are borderline, look for secondary signs such as meniscal extrusion, cartilage damage, subchondral BME, and parameniscal cysts.

- Be aware that the meniscus root attachments can have a normal striated appearance, specifically the anterior root of the LM, which must be differentiated from a tear.

DISCLOSURE

L.M. Trunz: Nothing to disclose. W.B. Morrison: -Medical Director/Founder, Trace Orthopedics, -Consultant, copatent owner, AprioMed, -Royalties, Elsevier, -Consultant, Zimmer-Biomet Inc, -Consultant, Medical Metrics Inc.

REFERENCES

1. Kim S, Bosque J, Meehan JP, et al. Increase in outpatient knee arthroscopy in the United States: a comparison of National Surveys of Ambulatory Surgery, 1996 and 2006. J Bone Joint Surg Am 2011; 93(11):994–1000.

2. Doral MN, Bilge O, Huri G, et al. Modern treatment of meniscal tears. EFORT Open Rev 2018;3(5):260–8.

3. Bhan K. Meniscal Tears: Current Understanding, Diagnosis, and Management. Cureus 2020;12(6): e8590.

4. Fox AJ, Bedi A, Rodeo SA. The basic science of human knee menisci: structure, composition, and function. Sports Health 2012;4(4):340–51.

5. Bryceland JK, Powell AJ, Nunn T. Knee Menisci Cartilage 2017;8(2):99–104.

6. Markes AR, Hodax JD, Ma CB. Meniscus Form and Function. Clin Sports Med 2020;39(1):1–12.

7. Tsujii A, Nakamura N, Horibe S. Age-related changes in the knee meniscus. Knee 2017;24(6): 1262–70.

8. Shahid S, Saghir N, Cawley O, et al. A Cadaveric Study of the Branching Pattern and Diameter of the Genicular Arteries: A Focus on the Middle Genicular Artery. J Knee Surg 2015;28(5):417–24.

9. Arnoczky SP, Warren RF. Microvasculature of the human meniscus. Am J Sports Med 1982;10(2):90–5.

10. Geffroy L. Meniscal pathology in children and adolescents. Orthop Traumatol Surg Res 2021; 107(1S):102775.

11. Pache S, Aman ZS, Kennedy M, et al. Meniscal Root Tears: Current Concepts Review. Arch Bone Jt Surg 2018;6(4):250–9.

12. Palisch AR, Winters RR, Willis MH, et al. Posterior Root Meniscal Tears: Preoperative, Intraoperative, and Postoperative Imaging for Transtibial Pullout Repair. Radiographics 2016;36(6):1792–806.

13. Kennedy MI, Strauss M, LaPrade RF. Injury of the Meniscus Root. Clin Sports Med 2020;39(1):57–68.

14. Gupte CM, Bull AM, Thomas RD, et al. A review of the function and biomechanics of the meniscofemoral ligaments. Arthroscopy 2003;19(2):161–71.

15. Knapik DM, Salata MJ, Voos JE, et al. Role of the Meniscofemoral Ligaments in the Stability of the Posterior Lateral Meniscus Root After Injury in the ACL-Deficient Knee. JBJS Rev 2020;8(1):e0071.

16. Mohankumar R, White LM, Naraghi A. Pitfalls and pearls in MRI of the knee. AJR Am J Roentgenol 2014;203(3):516–30.

17. De Maeseneer M, Van Roy F, Lenchik L, et al. Three layers of the medial capsular and supporting structures of the knee: MR imaging-anatomic correlation. Radiographics 2000;S83–9, 20 Spec No:.

18. Recondo JA, Salvador E, Villanúa JA, et al. Lateral stabilizing structures of the knee: functional anatomy and injuries assessed with MR imaging. Radiographics 2000;S91–102, 20 Spec No:.

19. Nguyen JC, De Smet AA, Graf BK, et al. MR imaging-based diagnosis and classification of meniscal tears. Radiographics 2014;34(4):981–99.

20. Nicholas JA. The five-one reconstruction for anteromedial instability of the knee. Indications, technique, and the results in fifty-two patients. J Bone Joint Surg Am 1973;55(5):899–922.

21. Smith JP 3rd, Barrett GR. Medial and lateral meniscal tear patterns in anterior cruciate ligament-deficient knees. A prospective analysis of 575 tears. Am J Sports Med 2001;29(4):415–9.

22. Vinson EN, Gage JA, Lacy JN. Association of peripheral vertical meniscal tears with anterior cruciate ligament tears. Skeletal Radiol 2008;37(7):645–51.

23. Vangsness CT Jr, DeCampos J, Merritt PO, et al. Meniscal injury associated with femoral shaft fractures. An arthroscopic evaluation of incidence. J Bone Joint Surg Br 1993;75(2):207–9.

24. Blacksin MF, Zurlo JV, Levy AS. Internal derangement of the knee after ipsilateral femoral shaft fracture: MR imaging findings. Skeletal Radiol 1998; 27(8):434–9.

25. Kocher MS, Micheli LJ, Gerbino P, et al. Tibial eminence fractures in children: prevalence of meniscal entrapment. Am J Sports Med 2003;31(3):404–7.

26. Rhodes JT, Cannamela PC, Cruz AI, et al. Incidence of Meniscal Entrapment and Associated Knee Injuries in Tibial Spine Avulsions. J Pediatr Orthop 2018;38(2):e38–42.

27. Lecouvet F, Van Haver T, Acid S, et al. Magnetic resonance imaging (MRI) of the knee: Identification of difficult-to-diagnose meniscal lesions. Diagn Interv Imaging 2018;99(2):55–64.

28. Shakoor D, Kijowski R, Guermazi A, et al. Diagnosis of Knee Meniscal Injuries by Using Three-dimensional MRI: A Systematic Review and Meta-Analysis of Diagnostic Performance. Radiology 2019;290(2):435–45.

29. Baker JC, Friedman MV, Rubin DA. Imaging the Postoperative Knee Meniscus: An Evidence-Based Review. AJR Am J Roentgenol 2018;211(3):519–27.

30. Morelli JN, Runge VM, Ai F, et al. An image-based approach to understanding the physics of MR artifacts. Radiographics 2011;31(3):849–66.

31. Fox MG, Graham JA, Skelton BW, et al. Prospective Evaluation of Agreement and Accuracy in the Diagnosis of Meniscal Tears: MR Arthrography a Short Time After Injection Versus CT Arthrography After a Moderate Delay. AJR Am J Roentgenol 2016; 207(1):142–9.

32. Lefevre N, Naouri JF, Herman S, et al. A Current Review of the Meniscus Imaging: Proposition of a Useful Tool for Its Radiologic Analysis. Radiol Res Pract 2016;2016:8329296.

33. Yaniv M, Blumberg N. The discoid meniscus. J Child Orthop 2007;1(2):89–96.

34. Samoto N, Kozuma M, Tokuhisa T, et al. Diagnosis of discoid lateral meniscus of the knee on MR imaging. Magn Reson Imaging 2002;20(1):59–64.

35. Mohankumar R, Palisch A, Khan W, et al. Meniscal ossicle: posttraumatic origin and association with posterior meniscal root tears. AJR Am J Roentgenol 2014;203(5):1040–6.

36. De Smet AA, Tuite MJ. Use of the "two-slice-touch" rule for the MRI diagnosis of meniscal tears. AJR Am J Roentgenol 2006;187(4):911–4.

37. Fritz B, Marbach G, Civardi F, et al. Deep convolutional neural network-based detection of meniscus tears: comparison with radiologists and surgery as standard of reference. Skeletal Radiol 2020;49(8): 1207–17.

38. De Smet AA. How I diagnose meniscal tears on knee MRI. AJR Am J Roentgenol 2012;199(3):481–99.

39. Alatakis S, Naidoo P. MR imaging of meniscal and cartilage injuries of the knee. Magn Reson Imaging Clin N Am 2009;17(4):741–756, vii.

40. Kijowski R, Rosas HG, Lee KS, et al. MRI characteristics of healed and unhealed peripheral vertical meniscal tears. AJR Am J Roentgenol 2014;202(3): 585–92.

41. Greif DN, Baraga MG, Rizzo MG, et al. MRI appearance of the different meniscal ramp lesion types, with clinical and arthroscopic correlation. Skeletal Radiol 2020;49(5):677–89.

42. Chahla J, Dean CS, Moatshe G, et al. Meniscal Ramp Lesions: Anatomy, Incidence, Diagnosis, and Treatment. Orthop J Sports Med 2016;4(7). 2325967116657815.

43. Davis KW, Rosas HG, Graf BK. Magnetic resonance imaging and arthroscopic appearance of the menisci of the knee. Clin Sports Med 2013;32(3): 449–75.

44. Anderson MW. MR imaging of the meniscus. Radiol Clin North Am 2002;40(5):1081–94.

45. Ridley WE, Xiang H, Han J, et al. Parrot beak and fish mouth signs: Meniscal tear. J Med Imaging Radiat Oncol 2018;62(Suppl 1):146–9485, 21_12786.

46. Gorbachova T, Melenevsky Y, Cohen M, et al. Osteochondral Lesions of the Knee: Differentiating the Most Common Entities at MRI. Radiographics 2018;38(5):1478–95.

47. Brody JM, Lin HM, Hulstyn MJ, et al. Lateral meniscus root tear and meniscus extrusion with anterior cruciate ligament tear. Radiology 2006; 239(3):805–10.

48. Kise NJ, Aga C, Engebretsen L, et al. Complex Tears, Extrusion, and Larger Excision Are Prognostic Factors for Worse Outcomes 1 and 2 Years After Arthroscopic Partial Meniscectomy for Degenerative Meniscal Tears: A Secondary Explorative Study of the Surgically Treated Group From the Odense-Oslo Meniscectomy Versus Exercise (OMEX) Trial. Am J Sports Med 2019;47(10):2402–11.

49. Dorsay TA, Helms CA. Bucket-handle meniscal tears of the knee: sensitivity and specificity of MRI signs. Skeletal Radiol 2003;32(5):266–72.

50. Bergin D, Hochberg H, Zoga AC, et al. Indirect soft-tissue and osseous signs on knee MRI of surgically proven meniscal tears. AJR Am J Roentgenol 2008; 191(1):86–92.

51. Costa CR, Morrison WB, Carrino JA. Medial meniscus extrusion on knee MRI: is extent associated with severity of degeneration or type of tear? AJR Am J Roentgenol 2004;183(1):17–23.

52. Carrino JA, Blum J, Parellada JA, et al. MRI of bone marrow edema-like signal in the pathogenesis of subchondral cysts. Osteoarthritis Cartil 2006; 14(10):1081–5.

53. Umans H, Morrison W, DiFelice GS, et al. Posterior horn medial meniscal root tear: the prequel. Skeletal Radiol 2014;43(6):775–80.

54. Hashimoto S, Terauchi M, Hatayama K, et al. Medial meniscus extrusion as a predictor for a poor prognosis in patients with spontaneous osteonecrosis of the knee. Knee 2021;31:164–71.

55. Campbell SE, Sanders TG, Morrison WB. MR imaging of meniscal cysts: incidence, location, and clinical significance. AJR Am J Roentgenol 2001; 177(2):409–13.

56. Beltran J, Marty-Delfaut E, Bencardino J, et al. Chondrocalcinosis of the hyaline cartilage of the knee: MRI manifestations. Skeletal Radiol 1998; 27(7):369–74.

57. Suan JC, Chhem RK, Gati JS, et al. 4 T MRI of chondrocalcinosis in combination with three-dimensional CT, radiography, and arthroscopy: a report of three cases. Skeletal Radiol 2005;34(11):714–21.

58. Kaushik S, Erickson JK, Palmer WE, et al. Effect of chondrocalcinosis on the MR imaging of knee menisci. AJR Am J Roentgenol 2001;177(4):905–9.

59. Park JS, Ryu KN, Yoon KH. Meniscal flounce on knee MRI: correlation with meniscal locations after positional changes. AJR Am J Roentgenol 2006; 187(2):364–70.

60. Wright RW, Boyer DS. Significance of the arthroscopic meniscal flounce sign: a prospective study. Am J Sports Med 2007;35(2):242–4.

61. Shankman S, Beltran J, Melamed E, et al. Anterior horn of the lateral meniscus: another potential pitfall in MR imaging of the knee. Radiology 1997;204(1): 181–4.

62. Feeley BT, Lau BC. Biomechanics and Clinical Outcomes of Partial Meniscectomy. J Am Acad Orthop Surg 2018;26(24):853–63.

63. Bansal S, Floyd ER, Kowalski MA, et al. Meniscal repair: The current state and recent advances in augmentation. J Orthop Res 2021;39(7):1368–82.

64. Tafur M, Probyn L, Chahal J, et al. Diagnosing Meniscal Pathology and Understanding How to Evaluate a Postoperative Meniscus Based on the Operative Procedure. J Knee Surg 2018;31(2): 166–83.

65. Yow BG, Donohue M, Tennent DJ. Meniscal Allograft Transplantation. Sports Med Arthrosc Rev 2021; 29(3):168–72.

Magnetic Resonance of Normal Variants of the Pediatric Knee

Hailey Allen, MD[a],*, Kirkland W. Davis, MD[b], Kara G. Gill, MD[b]

KEYWORDS

- Pediatric • Normal variant • Knee • Secondary ossification center • Discoid meniscus

KEY POINTS

- Review normal appearance of knee cartilage and bone marrow in children
- Discuss normal patterns of cartilage and physis maturation in the knee joint
- Discuss variations of bone and soft tissue structures found on magnetic resonance examinations of pediatric knees, including those that may be mistaken for pathollogy and those that may become symptomatic

INTRODUCTION

The interpretation of magnetic resonance (MR) imaging examinations of the knee joint in children brings with it unique challenges. Radiologists may be less comfortable with these studies because children undergo advanced imaging less frequently than adults. The physis, bone marrow, and cartilage of children also undergo significant changes over the course of skeletal maturation. Some variants of bone and cartilage may be difficult to distinguish from osteochondral pathology. Familiarity with the patterns of skeletal maturation and the most common and important variants seen on MR imaging can improve diagnostic confidence and help avoid misdiagnosis of pathology.

NORMAL MATURATION
Bone Marrow

At birth, bone marrow is dominated by hematopoietic elements. During the first year, conversion from hematopoietic marrow to fatty marrow in the appendicular skeleton begins in the epiphyses and ends in the metaphyses. Hematopoietic marrow may persist in long bone metaphyses into adulthood. Fatty marrow is hyperintense on T1-weighted images and hypointense with fat-suppression techniques. Hematopoietic marrow demonstrates intermediate signal intensity on T1-weighted images and intermediate to hyperintense signal on T2-weighted images. Hematopoietic marrow remains hyperintense relative to skeletal muscle on T1-weighted images because it still contains a significant proportion of fat cells (40% in hematopoietic marrow compared with 80% in fatty marrow).[1] Residual hematopoietic marrow in the long bone metaphyses of children may form flame-shaped patterns that abut the physis and show straight vertical margins. Discrete round islands of hematopoietic marrow also can be present.[2]

Epiphyseal Cartilage

In infants, the epiphyses, apophyses, and sesamoids are made of nonossified hyaline cartilage that matures via endochondral ossification. These cartilaginous structures appear isointense to muscle on T1-weighted images and hypointense on fluid-sensitive sequences.[2] In young children, the epiphyseal cartilage may be indistinguishable from the rim of articular cartilage forming along

a Department of Radiology & Imaging Sciences, University of Utah School of Medicine, 30 North 1900 East #1A071, Salt Lake City, UT 84132-2140, USA; b University of Wisconsin School of Medicine and Public Health, E3/366, 600 Highland Avenue, Madison, WI 53792-3252, USA
* Corresponding author.
E-mail address: Hailey.Allen@hsc.utah.edu

Magn Reson Imaging Clin N Am 30 (2022) 325–338
https://doi.org/10.1016/j.mric.2021.11.010

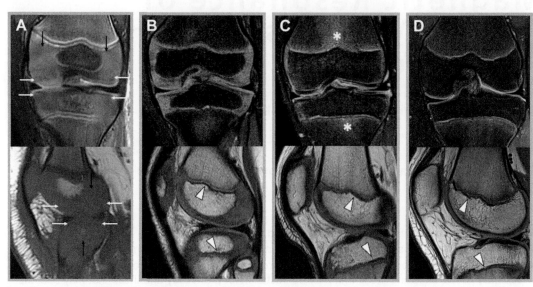

Fig. 1. (*A*) Coronal T2-weighted fat-suppressed (top) and sagittal T1-weighted (bottom) images in a 14-month-old boy. At early stages of skeletal maturation, it can be difficult to distinguish epiphyseal cartilage (*black arrows*) and articular cartilage (*white arrows*) due to their similar intensity on MR pulse sequences. Coronal T2-weighted (*top*) and sagittal proton density (PD) (*bottom*) MR images in a 5-year-old boy (*B*), 10-year-old boy (*C*), and 15-year-old boy (*D*) demonstrate normal progressive maturation of epiphyseal and articular cartilage. As the epiphysis ossifies, it becomes mineralized and populated with hematopoietic elements. At young ages, normal physes are wide and predominantly hyperintense in signal. Over time, the physis narrows and develops more distinct linear hypointense signal on its epiphyseal margin that corresponds to the ZPC (*white arrowheads*). Note residual T2 hyperintense hematopoietic elements within the metaphyses in the upper image of C (*asterisks*).

joint-facing margins (**Fig. 1**). Vascular channels may be identified within the periphery of unossified epiphyseal cartilage as thin tubular structures arranged in a spoke-wheel pattern. They may enhance following administration of intravenous contrast.[3] Epiphyseal ossification begins at centrally located spherical ossification centers that slowly increase in diameter and become populated by hematopoietic marrow. As epiphyseal ossification progresses, the subchondral bone plate appears and overlying hyaline articular cartilage assumes the adult shape and signal intensity. Secondary centers of ossification, common in the posterior femoral condyles and patella, are discussed later in the article.

Physis

The MR imaging appearance of the immature physis follows a standard pattern of development. In infancy, the physis is disk-shaped and uniformly wide. Three distinct layers are visible on MR imaging: a hyperintense layer on the epiphyseal side composed of the germinal, proliferative, and hypertrophic zones, a hypointense zone of provisional calcification (ZPC), and the vascular T2 hyperintense primary spongiosa on the metaphyseal side.[4,5] Over time, the physis becomes thinner and assumes an undulating contour, although its

trilaminar MR imaging appearance persists until physis closure (see **Fig. 1**). A thin hypointense physeal scar, thought to represent the remnant ZPC, is present in adolescents and young adults but eventually regresses.[2]

VARIANTS OF BONE AND CARTILAGE
Secondary Ossification Center of the Femur

A normal variant secondary ossification center (SOC) of the posterior femoral condyle is found in 66% of asymptomatic children. It is more common on the lateral side and is frequently bilateral.[6] On radiographs, SOCs appear as localized subchondral irregularity/spiculations involving the posterior weight-bearing femoral condyles. On MR imaging, the femoral SOC may show focally unossified cartilage with spiculated margins that can be hyperintense to the ossified epiphysis and distinct from the overlying hyaline articular cartilage (**Fig. 2**). Small ossicles may be present; these can be singular or multiple and can assume a round, "puzzle piece" or "incomplete puzzle piece" configuration.[7] Several features aid in distinguishing normal SOCs from osteochondritis dissecans (OCD) of the distal femur. SOCs are more common in younger patients (girls younger than 10 years and boys younger than 13), whereas OCDs are uncommon in patients younger than

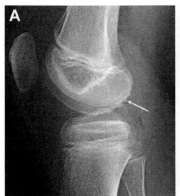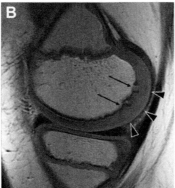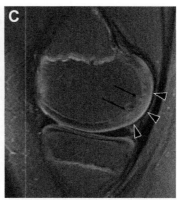

Fig. 2. An 11-year-old boy with knee pain. Lateral knee radiograph (*A*) shows irregularity of the posterior MFC (*white arrow*). Sagittal PD (*B*) and sagittal T2-weighted fat-suppressed (*C*) MR images demonstrate corresponding irregularity of the epiphyseal growth cartilage with spiculated margins (*black arrows*), overlain by intact articular cartilage (*black arrowheads*) and no associated bone marrow edema, consistent with a normal variant SOC.

8 years.[8] OCD classically involves the mesial or central femoral condyles and is more common medially (**Fig. 3**).[2] Disrupted articular cartilage, adjacent bone marrow edema, extension to the intercondylar notch, and undercutting fluid signal are more typical for OCD than SOC, whereas spiculations and multiple accessory ossifications are strongly associated with SOCs. Bilateral lesions, "puzzle piece" and "incomplete puzzle piece" ossifications can be present in both entities.[7,8] Distinguishing an SOC of the distal femur from OCD is important to ensure appropriate patient management and avoid unnecessary activity modifications and/or surgery.

Focal Periphyseal Edema Zone

MR examinations in adolescents with closing physes may reveal localized bone marrow edema radiating in a starburst pattern from the central physis into the adjacent epiphysis and metaphysis, known as a focal periphyseal edema (FOPE) zone (**Fig. 4**).[9] The physis at the center of a FOPE zone is not fused, although it may be narrowed. FOPE zones are believed to be caused by neovascularity and bleeding due to local stress and altered biomechanics occurring with impending physis closure, although the specific cause remains unknown. FOPE zones range in size from 2 to 27 mm in transverse dimension and are most evident on fluid-sensitive sequences in coronal or sagittal planes. They occur with similar incidence in the distal femur and proximal tibia but are rare elsewhere.[9] They are not typically associated with symptoms, although have been proposed as an etiology for knee pain in the absence of other abnormalities.[10] There is no radiographic correlate for FOPE zones, and they do not require further

workup or imaging follow-up. It is important not to mistake a FOPE zone for a physis injury or evidence of premature physis closure.

Bipartite Patella

Accessory ossification centers commonly form at the margins of the patella early in skeletal maturation.[11] Failure of accessory centers to fuse with the dominant ossification center can result in a bipartite patella or, less commonly, a tripartite/multipartite patella. Bipartite patella has a prevalence of 2% to 3% and is bilateral in 50% of cases.[12,13] In adolescence and adulthood, a bipartite patella appears as a well-corticated bone fragment of variable size that involves the superolateral quadrant 75% of the time. The overlying articular cartilage is usually intact and the synchondrosis lacks associated fluid signal or marrow edema; such cases are unlikely to cause symptoms (**Fig. 5**). Cases with marrow edema, fragmentation/fissuring of cartilage, or evidence of pseudoarthrosis may result in anterior pain that can improve with resection of the bipartite fragment.[13,14]

Dorsal Defect of the Patella

Dorsal defect of the patella (DDP) is a common variant typically identified radiographically as a well-circumscribed, round, lucent lesion in the superolateral patella. The DDP has a prevalence of up to 1%, although this may be an underestimate as the defects often resolve spontaneously in young adulthood.[12] DDP is bilateral in up to 33% of cases.[15] On MR imaging, a DDP arises from the subchondral bone plate of the superolateral patella. Adjacent bone marrow signal is typically normal. The overlying articular cartilage may be intact or may show central depression with

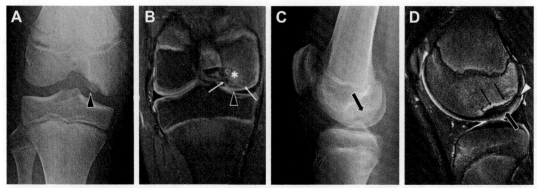

Fig. 3. Two patients with osteochondral lesions. Tunnel radiograph (A) in an 11-year-old boy with knee pain exacerbated by running. There is a curvilinear ossific fragment with corticated margins arising from the mesial aspect of the MFC (*black arrowhead*). Coronal T2-weighted fat-suppressed MR image (B) shows edema within the fragment (*black arrowhead*) and the adjacent femoral condyle marrow (*asterisk*). There is focal irregularity of the cartilage at the margins of the fragment and disruption of the subchondral bone plate (*white arrows*). This is unstable osteochondritis dissecans in a classic location. Lateral radiograph (C) in a 15-year-old boy with knee stiffness shows an osseous defect in the lateral femoral condyle (*block arrow*). Sagittal T2-weighted fat-suppressed MR image (D) shows marrow edema and fluid signal (*black arrows*) underlying the progeny fragment of an osteochondritis dissecans lesion (*block arrow*). There is disruption of the cartilage at the margin (*white arrowhead*), indicating likely instability. Both cases illustrate bone marrow edema and cartilage disruption, useful in differentiating osteochondral pathology from variant ossification centers.

focal hyperintense signal on fluid-sensitive sequences (**Fig. 6**).

Posterior Metaphyseal Stripe

A ubiquitous incidental finding on knee MR imaging in young patients is the posterior metaphyseal stripe. On its initial description by Laor and colleagues,[16] the posterior metaphyseal stripe was reported as a thin band of T2 hyperintense signal along the distal posterior metaphysis and was seen in all skeletally immature patients in the study as well as a portion of young adults (**Fig. 7**). Similar stripes are frequently visible in the posterior

proximal tibia. There is no radiographic correlate. Histologic analysis of the stripe reveals loose fibrovascular tissue, explaining enhancement of the stripe observed on postcontrast MR sequences. It is accepted as a normal and expected finding related to the significant growth occurring at the distal femur and proximal tibia.[2,16]

Distal Femur Cortical Irregularity

Also termed "cortical desmoid" and "distal femoral tug lesion," this variant is characterized by focal cortical irregularity/thickening, sometimes with concave or convex margins, at the distal posterior

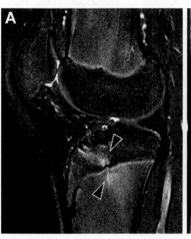
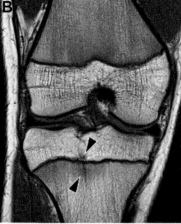

Fig. 4. A 14-year-old boy presenting with atraumatic knee pain. Sagittal T2-weighted fat-suppressed (A) and coronal T1-weighted (B) MR images demonstrate localized marrow edema radiating from the metaphyseal and epiphyseal sides of the centrally closing proximal tibial physis (*black arrowheads*), consistent with a FOPE zone. The absence of physis widening or intraphyseal fluid signal helps distinguish a FOPE zone from a physis injury.

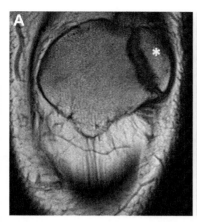
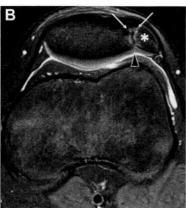

Fig. 5. A 15-year-old boy with chronic knee pain, exacerbated by playing football. Coronal T1-weighted (A) and axial PD fat-suppressed (B) MR images of the left knee demonstrate a bipartite patella. The superolateral quadrant of the patella gives rise to an independent osteochondral fragment with well-corticated margins (asterisks). In this case, the overlying articular cartilage is intact (black arrowhead) but there is focal bone marrow edema at the margins of the synchondrosis (white arrows), suggesting injury or chronic irritation to the synchondrosis of the bipartite patella.

medial femoral diaphysis.[17] It is an important "do not touch" lesion and should not be misinterpreted as aggressive periosteal reaction or parosteal osteosarcoma. On MR imaging, cortical irregularities manifest as irregularity at the site of attachment of the medial head of the gastrocnemius or tendon of the adductor magnus. The cortex typically shows normal hypointense signal with T2-hyperintense signal of the adjacent subcortical bone and a variably present thin sclerotic rim (**Fig. 8**). Acute injury or chronic repetitive traction may result in edema within the tendon attachment or of the surrounding tissues.[18]

Inferior Pole Fragmentation of the Patella

Small linear or crescent-shaped corticated ossific fragments at the inferior pole of the patella in young children have been posited to represent variant centers of ossification. However, the increasing use of MR imaging has shown such ossifications are frequently associated with marrow edema and/or abnormal surrounding fluid signal, suggesting the finding is more likely related to avulsion injury or repetitive stress, comprising part of the pathologic spectrum including patellar sleeve avulsion and Sinding-Larsen-Johansson disease (**Fig. 9**).[19]

MENISCUS AND LIGAMENT VARIANTS
Discoid Meniscus

Discoid meniscus (DM) is the most common developmental variant of the knee joint in children, with an incidence of 0.4% to 17%.[20,21] DM much more commonly affects the lateral meniscus. Rather

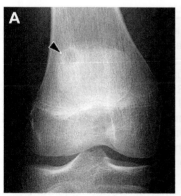
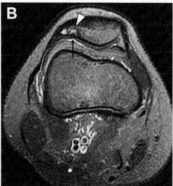
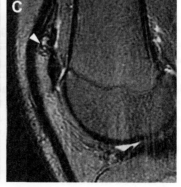

Fig. 6. A 14-year-old girl injured playing soccer. Anteroposterior radiograph of the knee (A) shows a lucent round lesion within the superolateral quadrant of the patella (black arrowhead), consistent with a DDP. Axial (B) and sagittal (C) T2-weighted fat-suppressed MR images confirm the well-circumscribed defect in the subchondral bone of the superolateral patella (white arrowheads). In this case, the articular cartilage that fills the defect (black arrow in B) is slightly thinner and more hyperintense than the cartilage elsewhere.

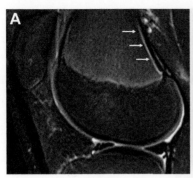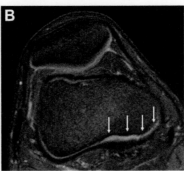

Fig. 7. A 14-year-old boy with knee pain after a fall. Sagittal T2-weighted fat-suppressed (*A*) and axial PD fat-suppressed (*B*) MR images demonstrate a thin layer of T2 hyperintense signal (*white arrows*) subjacent to the posterior metaphyseal cortex, commensurate with a normal posterior metaphyseal stripe. The absence of cortical thickening distinguishes this finding from the distal femur cortical irregularity/cortical desmoid, which also occurs in this location.

than being a normal C-shape, a DM has an abnormally thickened outer rim and is completely filled in centrally or has only a small void (**Fig. 10**). On MR imaging, DM is diagnosed when there are 3 or more contiguous sagittal images demonstrating continuity between the anterior and posterior horns.[20,22]

The Watanabe classification describes DM as complete (type 1), incomplete (type 2), or Wrisberg type (type 3). Type 1 is most common, with the thickened lateral meniscus filling the entire lateral compartment. Type 2 covers less than 80% of the lateral tibial plateau and has concave inner margins. Both types 1 and 2 maintain normal peripheral attachments. A type 3 meniscus may be discoid or C-shaped but lacks the normal posterior meniscus attachments. The hypermobile type 3 DM may subluxate anteriorly during flexion and reduce with a clunk during extension, a condition known as "snapping knee syndrome."[20,21] It may also migrate into the intercondylar notch, resulting in a "pseudo-bucket-handle tear." Unlike a true bucket-handle meniscus tear (BHMT), there should be no residual meniscus tissue at the periphery.[20]

DMs are predisposed to early degeneration and tearing.[21] Shape deformation, increased intrameniscal signal, or both can signify a tear in the setting of DM, especially in a symptomatic pediatric patient. The intrameniscal signal need not be linear.[20] Younger patients with DM tears typically present with popping or snapping, whereas older children more commonly report acute pain, locking, or inability to bear weight.[20,21]

Ring-Shaped Meniscus

Ring-shaped meniscus (RSM) results when there is a bridge of meniscus tissue between the anterior and posterior horns of the medial or lateral meniscus that forms a complete ring. On mid-

coronal images, the triangular intermeniscal bridge is visible as a mirror image of the meniscus body, known as the "mirror image sign" (**Fig. 11**). The bridge is differentiated from a BHMT by its smooth triangular shape and the normal morphology of the meniscus body.[23,24] RSM is asymptomatic unless torn and can be associated with congenital hypoplasia or absence of the anterior cruciate ligament.[24]

Meniscal Flounce

Meniscal flounce is a normal variant related to transient distortion of the inner margin of the medial meniscus that may be due to patient positioning. The wavy contour or single fold along the free edge of the meniscus is best identified on sagittal images (**Fig. 12**). On coronal images, the meniscus free edge may appear truncated due to volume averaging, mimicking a radial tear. However, there is no corresponding meniscus defect or signal abnormality on sagittal images.[25–27]

Meniscal Ossicle

Meniscal ossicles are small foci of ossification within the posterior horn of the medial meniscus. Although some result from dystrophic ossification due to prior trauma, others may be developmental variants. On MR imaging, meniscal ossicles have a rim of cortical bone and central marrow fat (**Fig. 13**). Intra-articular bodies from osteochondral fractures or synovial chondromatosis can have similar signal characteristics but are not intrameniscal in location.[25,28]

Triple-Bundle Anterior Cruciate Ligament

Traditional understanding of anterior cruciate ligament (ACL) anatomy is that there are 2 major bundles, anteromedial (AM) and posterolateral (PL), which together restrain anterior tibial translation.

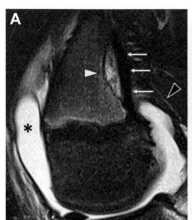
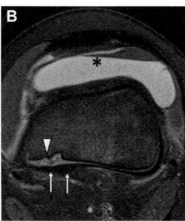

Fig. 8. A 12-year-old girl presenting with knee pain after an injury. Sagittal T2-weighted fat-suppressed (A) and axial PD fat-suppressed (B) MR images show focal thickening of the posterior metaphyseal cortex of the distal femur (*white arrows*) with a subjacent well-circumscribed T2-hyperintense lesion with lobulated margins and a thin sclerotic border (*white arrowheads*). The location coincides with the origin of the medial head of the gastrocnemius (*black arrowhead*). This imaging appearance is typical for distal femur cortical irregularity. The large lipohemarthrosis (*asterisks*) is due to an acute tibia fracture (not shown).

Recent publications document a third bundle, the intermediate (IM) bundle, in some patients. True prevalence is unknown, but one MR study documented an IM bundle, whether complete or partial (beginning distal to the femoral origin of the ACL), in 15 of 73 MR scans.[29] The IM bundle projects anterior to and between the AM and PL bundles, with normal low signal (**Fig. 14**).[29] Function and importance of this structure remain speculative.[25]

ABSENT/HYPOPLASTIC ANTERIOR CRUCIATE LIGAMENT

Although the ACL is often absent or hypoplastic in patients with major limb developmental deformities such as proximal femoral focal deficiency,

fibular hemimelia, or thrombocytopenia-absent radius syndrome, absent ACL may be an isolated condition.[30,31] Posterior cruciate ligament (PCL) deficiency may accompany ACL aplasia but does not occur on its own.[31] Developmental deficiency of the ACL may lead to instability, pain, cartilage loss, and meniscus tears; however, patients may also adapt to their instability and remain relatively symptom-free.[30] In older patients with no ACL, the question may arise whether the patient suffered a remote ACL rupture or just developed without one. The answer is found in the bone morphology: the developmentally deficient ACL results in dysplasia of the femur and tibia. Specifically, the intercondylar notch will be narrower or shallower, the tibial spines will be smoother and

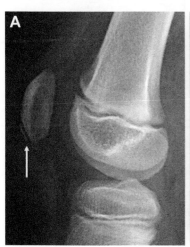
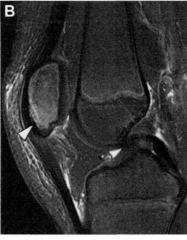

Fig. 9. An 11-year-old boy presenting with pain at and below the patella from a soccer injury. (A) Lateral radiograph of the knee shows linear ossified fragments at the anteroinferior margin of the patella (*white arrow*). (B) Sagittal T2-weighted fat-suppressed MR image of the knee shows bone marrow edema localized to the inferior patella (*white arrowhead*) with peripatellar soft tissue swelling and edema in Hoffa fat pad. This site has been posited to be a center of secondary ossification like the posterior femoral condyles; however, studies incorporating MR imaging and clinical data suggest

that fragmentation at the inferior pole is more likely to be related to sleeve avulsion at the inferior pole rather than normal variation.

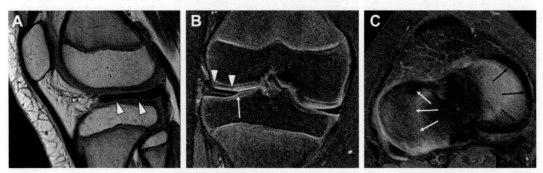

Fig. 10. A 10-year-old boy with knee pain. Sagittal PD (*A*), coronal PD fat-suppressed (*B*), and axial PD fat-suppressed (*C*) images of the right knee demonstrate a disk-shaped, thickened, globular LM consistent with a DM (*white arrowheads*). The free edge of the lateral meniscal body extends past the midpoint of the lateral compartment (*white arrows*), in comparison with the normal thin, C-shaped MM (*black arrows*). Because this meniscus does not cover the entire lateral compartment, it is classified as an incomplete (type 2) DM.

smaller, the tibial plateau may become convex superiorly, and the femoral condyles are flatter (**Fig. 15**).[32,33] The dysplastic changes are more severe if the ACL is absent as opposed to hypoplastic; and even more so if the PCL is diminutive or absent.[31]

MENISCOFEMORAL LIGAMENTS

The meniscofemoral ligaments (MFL) have been well known pitfalls since the early days of knee MR.[34] These structures connect the posterior horn of the lateral meniscus (LM) to the medial femoral condyle (MFC) at the intercondylar notch.

The MFLs hold the LM in a constant position throughout the range of motion.[35] The MFL of Humphry passes anterior to the PCL and the MFL of Wrisberg passes posterior to the PCL (**Fig. 16**), although MFLs may also attach to the PCL directly.[36] As cadaver, surgical, and MR estimates of percentages of knees that exhibit one or both MFLs vary widely, note that it is typical to see one MFL or the other on MR but to see both is uncommon.[36,37] Common pitfalls are mistaking the junction of an MFL and the LM for a meniscus tear and misinterpreting a portion of an MFL for an intra-articular body.

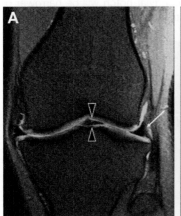
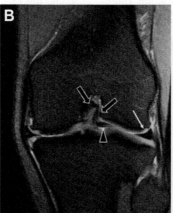
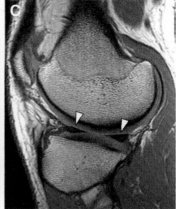

Fig. 11. A 19-year-old female soccer player presenting with worsening knee instability. Coronal PD fat-suppressed MR images (*A, B*) show a triangular hypointense structure (*black arrowheads*) that was continuous anteriorly and posteriorly with the anterior and posterior horns of the LM. Initially, this was thought to be a bucket-handle tear of the LM, but the lateral meniscal body (*white arrow*) was intact and appears normal. Note the otherwise normal morphology of the anterior and posterior horns (*white arrowheads*) on the sagittal PD MR image (*C*), confirming an RSM. The patient lacked a normal ACL but was found to have a variant thin ligamentous structure extending from the superomedial intercondylar notch to the posterior aspect of the ring meniscus (*black arrows*). Surgery confirmed the MR findings.

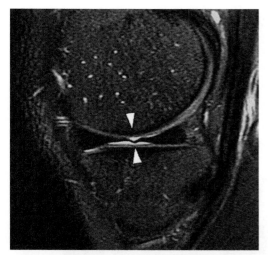

Fig. 12. Sagittal T2-weighted MR image in an 18-year-old man with an incidentally noted meniscal flounce (*white arrowheads*). There is focal redundancy and undulation of the body of the MM. No meniscus tear was present.

Anteromedial Meniscofemoral Ligament

A recently described but uncommon (<1%) variation is the anteromedial (AM) MFL. This structure arises near the ACL origin in the intercondylar notch and descends anterior to the ACL at the same or slightly shallower angle.[38,39] In the original description, it inserts into the anterior horn/root of the medial meniscus (MM), although the current authors and others note its predominant insertion is the medial aspect of the transverse intermeniscal ligament. It appears as a thin low-signal band and may mimic the infrapatellar plica[37]; the difference is that the plica extends farther anteriorly and inserts into Hoffa fat pad (**Fig. 17**). The AMMFL can be distinguished from a longitudinal split tear of the

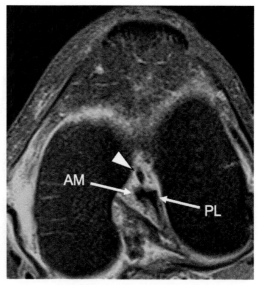

Fig. 14. A 36-year-old woman with knee pain after a fall while skiing. Axial PD fat-suppressed MR image of the inferior intercondylar notch shows a variant third bundle of the ACL (*white arrowhead*) coursing anterior to the typical anteromedial (AM) and posterolateral (PL) bundles (*white arrows*).

ACL by the AMMFL's insertion onto the MM or intermeniscal ligament.

OBLIQUE MENISCOMENISCAL LIGAMENT

An oblique meniscomeniscal ligament (OMML) is present on 1% to 4% of knee MRs. This low-signal collagenous band attaches the anterior horn of one meniscus to the posterior horn of the other and is named based on which meniscus is its anterior attachment (**Fig. 18**).[37,40] This variant has no known function but should not be mistaken

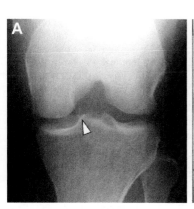
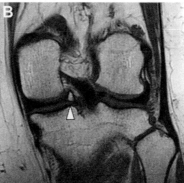

Fig. 13. A 25-year-old woman with mild knee pain after an injury. (*A*) Tunnel view radiograph of the knee shows a well-corticated ossified fragment adjacent to the medial tibial spine (*white arrowhead*). (*B*) Coronal T1-weighted MR image shows the ossified fragment (*white arrowhead*) to be associated with the posterior horn of the MM. The fragment is identical in signal intensity to normal bone, without sclerosis or edema. This is a meniscal ossicle. Although a congenital origin has been proposed, due to a high association with meniscus tears, many meniscal ossicles are considered posttraumatic or degenerative in origin.

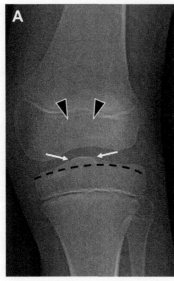
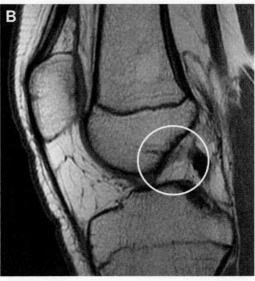

Fig. 15. A 9-year-old girl with bilateral knee pain. Anteroposterior radiograph of the left knee (*A*) reveals morphologic findings characteristic of congenital absence of the ACL. The tibial eminence is smooth with diminutive tibial spines (*white arrows*). The tibial plateau is convex superiorly (*dashed line*), and the intercondylar notch is narrow (*black arrowheads*). Sagittal PD MR image (*B*) of the same patient at age 15 confirms an absent ACL (*circle*).

for pathology such as a BHMT. The key to recognizing the OMML as a normal structure instead of a BHMT is that neither meniscus will be missing the central portion as is seen with true BHMT.[37]

ACCESSORY MUSCLES

Several accessory or anomalous muscles have been described about the knee joint and can be identified on MR imaging. There are multiple variants involving the gastrocnemius muscle. The most common of these is the third head of the gastrocnemius, also called gastrocnemius tertius, with an incidence of 2.9% to 5.5%.[41] The third

head ranges in size from a thin cord of muscle to a large muscular head like the medial or lateral heads. It arises near the midline along the posterior distal femur, lies posterolateral to the popliteal vessels, and joins distally with either the medial or lateral head of the gastrocnemius. Accessory slips of the gastrocnemius may arise from either the medial or lateral head. An accessory slip of the medial gastrocnemius originates from the intercondylar notch, courses between the popliteal artery and vein, and inserts into the distal medial head. An accessory slip of the lateral gastrocnemius originates from the posterior femur above and medial to the lateral head, lies deep to the

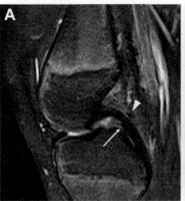
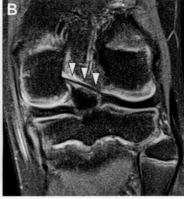

Fig. 16. An 11-year-old boy with knee pain after a fall. Sagittal T2-weighted fat-suppressed (*A*) and coronal PD fat-suppressed (*B*) MR images show normal meniscofemoral ligaments coursing from the posterior horn of the LM to the lateral aspect of the MFC within the intercondylar notch. The meniscofemoral ligament of Humphry (*white arrow*) passes anterior to the PCL. The meniscofemoral ligament of Wrisberg (*white arrowheads*) passes posterior to the PCL. The meniscofemoral ligament of Wrisberg is more prevalent and tends to be more robust than Humphry.

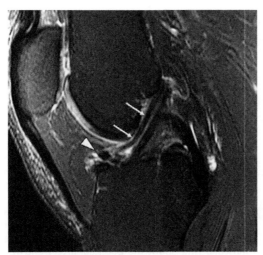

Fig. 17. A 57-year-old woman with chronic knee pain explained by cartilage loss and MM tear (not shown). Sagittal fat-suppressed T2-weighted MR image demonstrates an AMMFL (*white arrows*). The AMMFL originates from the lateral wall of the intercondylar notch and inserts onto the anterior horn of the MM. In this case, its insertion is partially onto the transverse intermeniscal ligament (*white arrowhead*), as well as the MM.

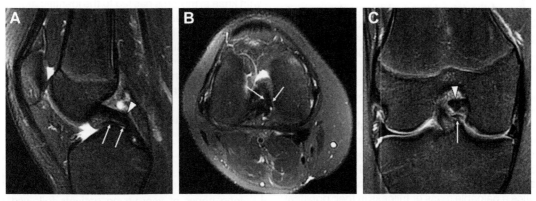

Fig. 18. A 14-year-old girl with knee pain and concern for meniscus tear. Sagittal T2-weighted fat-suppressed MR image (*A*) shows a low-signal band (*white arrows*) just below the PCL (*white arrowheads*), which might be mistaken for a double PCL sign from a BHMT. Instead, this is a lateral OMML. The "lateral" designation means that it attaches to the anterior horn of the LM and the posterior horn of the MM. Axial T2-weighted fat-suppressed (*B*) and coronal PD fat-suppressed MR images (*C*) show the OMML (*white arrows*) extending obliquely across the tibial eminence and lying inferior to the PCL (*white arrowhead*).

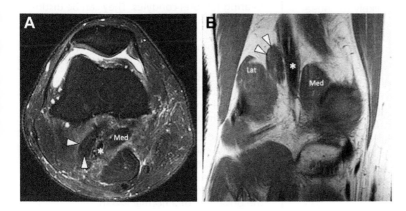

Fig. 19. A 43-year-old man with chronic knee pain. Axial T2-weighted fat-suppressed (*A*) and coronal PD (*B*) MR images show an extra muscle within the popliteal fossa (*white arrowheads*) at the medial margin of the lateral head of the gastrocnemius (Lat). This is an accessory slip of the lateral head of the gastrocnemius, which in combination with the medial head of the gastrocnemius (Med), forms a muscular ring around the popliteal neurovascular bundle (*asterisk*).

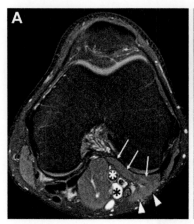 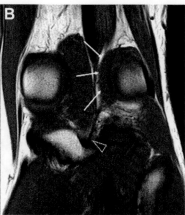

Fig. 20. A 24-year-old man with knee pain after an injury. Axial PD fat-suppressed (*A*) and coronal T1-weighted (*B*) MR images show an accessory muscle within the deep lateral aspect of the popliteal fossa (*white arrows*). Proximally this muscle arises together with the lateral head of the gastrocnemius (*white arrowheads*) and distally the muscle inserts onto the posteromedial joint capsule (*black arrowhead*), as is typical for an accessory popliteus muscle. In combination with the medial and lateral heads of the gastrocnemius, the accessory popliteus forms a muscular ring about the popliteal artery and vein (*white* and *black asterisks*, respectively).

popliteal vessels, and inserts on the distal lateral head (**Fig. 19**).[42]

The accessory popliteus arises at the medial margin of the lateral head of the gastrocnemius above the normal popliteus muscle. It passes obliquely through the popliteal fossa, deep to the neurovascular structures, to insert on the posteromedial joint capsule (**Fig. 20**).[43]

The tensor fasciae suralis is a rare variant located superficially within the popliteal fossa with variable length and inconsistent attachments. It originates from the distal hamstring muscles, typically the semitendinosus, and inserts into the Achilles tendon or less commonly onto the superficial fascia of the leg or medial head of the gastrocnemius.[44,45] Patients with this variant may notice a palpable mass or fullness in their popliteal fossa, although most cases remain asymptomatic.

The accessory plantaris is a small but common variant, appreciated in 6.3% of knee MR images in one study. It arises from the plantaris muscle and inserts proximally into the iliotibial band or lateral retinaculum. Its small size and superficial/lateral location make this variant unlikely to cause symptoms.[46]

The medial and lateral accessory slips of the gastrocnemius and the accessory popliteus form muscular rings about the popliteal vessels and can result in compression of the popliteal artery with plantar flexion or dorsiflexion, known as popliteal artery entrapment syndrome. Typical patients with entrapment syndrome are active young adults with leg claudication. Functional evaluation of patients with predisposing muscle variants can be performed with dynamic MR angiography. The third head of the gastrocnemius, tensor fasciae suralis, and accessory plantaris do not encircle the popliteal vessels and are unlikely to cause entrapment.[42,44]

SUMMARY

The increasing utilization of MR imaging in children with knee symptoms has led to the identification of numerous developmental or congenital variants, some of which may be mistaken for pathology. An understanding of features distinguishing normal variants from true abnormalities is essential to accurate diagnosis and the avoidance of unnecessary treatment.

CLINICS CARE POINTS

- Hematopoietic marrow predominates in the long bones of very young patients followed by a patterned conversion to fatty marrow. Flame-shaped or vertically striated residual hematopoietic elements may be present in the metaphyses of adolescents and young adults.

- Normal variant secondary ossification centers frequently occur at the posterior weight-bearing femoral condyles. They can be distinguished from osteochondritis dissecans by their posterior location, the presence of spiculated margins, intact overlying articular cartilage, and the absence of marrow edema.

- DM is a common variant that predisposes to meniscus degeneration and tears. The absence of normal posterior attachments may suggest meniscal hypermobility/instability.

- Subluxated DM, RSM, and numerous variant ligaments can be mistaken for bucket-handle meniscal tears. In the absence of defect in the known normal structures of the knee or substantial adjacent edema, one should consider the possibility of a normal variant.

DISCLOSURE

The authors have no relevant conflicts of interest to disclose.

REFERENCES

1. Vogler JB 3rd, Murphy WA. Bone marrow imaging. Radiology 1988;168(3):679–93.
2. Laor T, Jaramillo D. MR imaging insights into skeletal maturation: what is normal? Radiology 2009;250(1):28–38.
3. Chung SM. The arterial supply of the developing proximal end of the human femur. J Bone Joint Surg Am 1976;58(7):961–70.
4. Yun HH, Kim HJ, Jeong MS, et al. Changes of the growth plate in children: 3-dimensional magnetic resonance imaging analysis. Korean J Pediatr 2018;61(7):226–30.
5. Jaramillo D, Connolly SA, Mulkern RV, et al. Developing epiphysis: MR imaging characteristics and histologic correlation in the newborn lamb. Radiology 1998;207(3):637–45.
6. Caffey J, Madell SH, Royer C, et al. Ossification of the distal femoral epiphysis. J Bone Joint Surg Am 1958;40-A(3):647–54. passim.
7. Gebarski K, Hernandez RJ. Stage-I osteochondritis dissecans versus normal variants of ossification in the knee in children. Pediatr Radiol 2005;35(9):880–6.
8. Jans LB, Jaremko JL, Ditchfield M, et al. MRI differentiates femoral condylar ossification evolution from osteochondritis dissecans. A new sign. Eur Radiol 2011;21(6):1170–9.
9. Zbojniewicz AM, Laor T. Focal periphyseal edema (FOPE) zone on MRI of the adolescent knee: a potentially painful manifestation of physiologic physeal fusion? AJR Am J Roentgenol 2011;197(4):998–1004.
10. Gilos E, Nicholson A, Sharkey MS, et al. Focal periphyseal edema: are we overtreating physiologic adolescent knee pain? J Am Acad Orthop Surg Glob Res Rev 2018;2(4):e047.
11. Ogden JA. Radiology of postnatal skeletal development. X. Patella and tibial tuberosity. Skeletal Radiol 1984;11(4):246–57.
12. van Holsbeeck M, Vandamme B, Marchal G, et al. Dorsal defect of the patella: concept of its origin and relationship with bipartite and multipartite patella. Skeletal Radiol 1987;16(4):304–11.
13. Vaz A, Trippia CR. Small but troublesome: accessory ossicles with clinical significance. Radiol Bras 2018;51(4):248–56.
14. Kavanagh EC, Zoga A, Omar I, et al. MRI findings in bipartite patella. Skeletal Radiol 2007;36(3):209–14.
15. Ho VB, Kransdorf MJ, Jelinek JS, et al. Dorsal defect of the patella: MR features. J Comput Assist Tomogr 1991;15(3):474–6.
16. Laor T, Chun GF, Dardzinski BJ, et al. Posterior distal femoral and proximal tibial metaphyseal stripes at MR imaging in children and young adults. Radiology 2002;224(3):669–74.
17. Resnick D, Greenway G. Distal femoral cortical defects, irregularities, and excavations. Radiology 1982;143(2):345–54.
18. Vieira RL, Bencardino JT, Rosenberg ZS, et al. MRI features of cortical desmoid in acute knee trauma. AJR Am J Roentgenol 2011;196(2):424–8.
19. Kan JH, Vogelius ES, Orth RC, et al. Inferior patellar pole fragmentation in children: just a normal variant? Pediatr Radiol 2015;45(6):882–7.
20. Restrepo R, Weisberg MD, Pevsner R, et al. Discoid meniscus in the pediatric population:: emphasis on MR imaging signs of instability. Magn Reson Imaging Clin N Am 2019;27(2):323–39.
21. Kushare I, Klingele K, Samora W. Discoid meniscus: diagnosis and management. Orthop Clin North Am 2015;46(4):533–40.
22. Thapa MM, Chaturvedi A, Iyer RS, et al. MRI of pediatric patients: part 2, normal variants and abnormalities of the knee. AJR Am J Roentgenol 2012;198(5):W456–65.
23. Iqbal A, McLoughlin E, Botchu R, et al. The ring-shaped meniscus: a case series demonstrating the variation of imaging appearances on MRI. Skeletal Radiol 2020;49(2):281–9.
24. Esteves C, Castro R, Cadilha R, et al. Ring-shaped lateral meniscus with hypoplasic anterior cruciate ligament. Skeletal Radiol 2015;44(12):1813–8.
25. Tan K, Yoong P, Toms AP. Normal anatomical variants of the menisci and cruciate ligaments that may mimic disease. Clin Radiol 2014;69(11):1178–85.
26. Yu JS, Cosgarea AJ, Kaeding CC, et al. Meniscal flounce MR imaging. Radiology 1997;203(2):513–5.
27. Park JS, Ryu KN, Yoon KH. Meniscal flounce on knee MRI: correlation with meniscal locations after positional changes. AJR Am J Roentgenol 2006;187(2):364–70.
28. Schnarkowski P, Tirman PF, Fuchigami KD, et al. Meniscal ossicle: radiographic and MR imaging findings. Radiology 1995;196(1):47–50.
29. MacKay JW, Whitehead H, Toms AP. Radiological evidence for the triple bundle anterior cruciate ligament. Clin Anat 2014;27(7):1097–102.
30. Ergun S, Karahan M, Akgun U, et al. [A case of multiple congenital anomalies including agenesis of the anterior cruciate ligament]. Acta Orthop Traumatol Turc 2008;42(5):373–6. On capraz bag agenezisini de iceren coklu dogustan anomalili bir olgu.
31. Manner HM, Radler C, Ganger R, et al. Dysplasia of the cruciate ligaments: radiographic assessment and classification. J Bone Joint Surg Am 2006;88(1):130–7.
32. Balke M, Mueller-Huebenthal J, Shafizadeh S, et al. Unilateral aplasia of both cruciate ligaments. J Orthop Surg Res 2010;5:11.

33. Bedoya MA, McGraw MH, Wells L, et al. Bilateral agenesis of the anterior cruciate ligament: MRI evaluation. Pediatr Radiol 2014;44(9):1179–83.

34. Herman LJ, Beltran J. Pitfalls in MR imaging of the knee. Radiology 1988;167(3):775–81.

35. Poynton A, Moran CJ, Moran R, et al. The meniscofemoral ligaments influence lateral meniscal motion at the human knee joint. Arthroscopy 2011;27(3):365–71.

36. Cho JM, Suh JS, Na JB, et al. Variations in meniscofemoral ligaments at anatomical study and MR imaging. Skeletal Radiol 1999;28(4):189–95.

37. Tyler P, Datir A, Saifuddin A. Magnetic resonance imaging of anatomical variations in the knee. Part 1: ligamentous and musculotendinous. Skeletal Radiol 2010;39(12):1161–73.

38. Alves T, Braun MAA, Duarte ML, et al. Anteromedial meniscofemoral ligament—A rare finding. Morphologie 2021. https://doi.org/10.1016/j.morpho.2021.03.004.

39. Liu YW, Skalski MR, Patel DB, et al. The anterior knee: normal variants, common pathologies, and diagnostic pitfalls on MRI. Skeletal Radiol 2018; 47(8):1069–86.

40. Kim HK, Laor T. Oblique meniscomeniscal ligament: a normal variant. Pediatr Radiol Jun 2009;39(6):634.

41. Koplas MC, Grooff P, Piraino D, et al. Third head of the gastrocnemius: an MR imaging study based on 1,039 consecutive knee examinations. Skeletal Radiol 2009;38(4):349–54.

42. Sookur PA, Naraghi AM, Bleakney RR, et al. Accessory muscles: anatomy, symptoms, and radiologic evaluation. Radiographics 2008;28(2):481–99.

43. Duc SR, Wentz KU, Kach KP, et al. First report of an accessory popliteal muscle: detection with MRI. Skeletal Radiol 2004;33(7):429–31.

44. Chason DP, Schultz SM, Fleckenstein JL. Tensor fasciae suralis: depiction on MR images. AJR Am J Roentgenol 1995;165(5):1220–1.

45. Tubbs RS, Salter EG, Oakes WJ. Dissection of a rare accessory muscle of the leg: the tensor fasciae suralis muscle. Clin Anat 2006;19(6):571–2.

46. Herzog RJ. Accessory plantaris muscle: anatomy and prevalence. HSS J Feb 2011;7(1):52–6.

Intra-articular Neoplasms and Masslike Lesions of the Knee: Emphasis on MR Imaging

Adam Rudd, MD*, Mini N. Pathria, MD

KEYWORDS

- Knee • MR imaging • Intra-articular neoplasm • Pigmented villonodular synovitis
- Primary synovial chondromatosis • Synovial hemangioma

KEY POINTS

- Distinguishing between intra-articular knee masses that present as a diffuse/multifocal process and that of a focal mass is useful in narrowing the differential diagnosis.
- Some entities have a diffuse and a focal form, such as pigmented villonodular synovitis and focal nodular synovitis.
- The MR imaging features are often pathognomonic. However, CT and plain radiography are useful adjunctive modalities to better demonstrate calcification within masses and extrinsic osseous erosions, which can easily be overlooked at MR imaging.

INTRODUCTION

Intra-articular masses of the knee joint encompass a diverse group of entities that include neoplastic and nonneoplastic proliferative lesions that can affect the articulation diffusely, produce multiple disseminated lesions, or present as a discrete solitary mass. MR imaging plays an integral role in the identification and characterization of joint disorders because of its high spatial resolution and excellent soft tissue contrast. Although some intra-articular masses have distinct MR imaging findings that allow confident diagnosis, many are nonspecific and require biopsy for final diagnosis. This article focuses on the most common primary articular disorders that present as an intra-articular mass, with an emphasis on their characteristic MR imaging features. Extra-articular masses and masslike lesions related to infection, systemic inflammatory arthritis, and deposition disorders are discussed elsewhere in this issue.

SPECIFIC NEOPLASMS

The imaging diagnosis of an intraarticular mass of the knee relies on the age of the patient, the geographic distribution of the mass within the joint, and its specific imaging features. It is helpful to categorize knee masses into those that are diffuse/multifocal entities that generally parallel the distribution of the articular synovial lining versus those that appear solitary, presenting as a focal mass within only a portion of the joint.

Diffuse/Multifocal Neoplasms

Primary synovial chondromatosis

Primary synovial chondromatosis (PSC) is an uncommon disorder characterized by the formation of multiple foci of benign hyaline cartilage within the subsynovial tissue of a joint, tendon sheath, or bursa.[1,2] The knee is the most commonly involved joint, comprising approximately 50% to 65% of cases.[1] These chondral foci can enlarge, detach from the synovium to become intra-articular, and eventually ossify. Secondary synovial osteochondromatosis, referring to multiple osteochondral bodies within a diseased joint, is a far more common entity than PSC. The secondary form is usually secondary to advanced osteoarthrosis but may also be seen in the setting of trauma, osteochondritis dissecans, neuropathic osteoarthropathy, or prior joint

Department of Radiology, UCSD Health System, University of California, HCOP MRI, 408 Dickinson Street, San Diego, CA 92103-8226, USA
* Corresponding author.
E-mail address: Arudd689@gmail.com

Magn Reson Imaging Clin N Am 30 (2022) 339–350
https://doi.org/10.1016/j.mric.2021.11.011

infection.[1] PSC is differentiated from secondary synovial osteochondromatosis by the presence of a greater number of bodies of more uniform size evenly distributed throughout a joint that otherwise appears normal (**Fig. 1**).

The treatment of choice for PSC is removal of the chondral fragments with or without synovectomy. Multiple recurrences or the development of marrow invasion should raise concern for malignant transformation,[1] a rare complication of PSC. Malignant transformation to chondrosarcoma is reported to occur in 2.5% of patients, most commonly at the hip joint.[2] These chondrosarcomas are typically low-grade, locally aggressive tumors that do not give rise to metastases.[2]

When mineralized, the imaging features of PSC are often pathognomonic on radiographs and computed tomography (CT), demonstrating the characteristic ring and arc calcification typical of ossifying cartilage. Calcifications are present in 70% to 95% of cases and are typically distributed widely throughout the synovium.[1,3] CT offers an advantage over radiography for the detection of extrinsic osseous erosions, which occur in 20% to 50%.[1] MR imaging findings are variable depending on the amount of mineralization of the foci of cartilage. Kramer and colleagues[4] described three distinct MR imaging patterns in patients with surgically proven PSC. The most common pattern, seen in 77% of patients, was characterized by lobulated, homogeneous, intra-articular signal that was isointense to slightly hyperintense to skeletal muscle on T1-weighted images and hyperintense on T2-weighted images with recognizable foci of hypointense calcifications (**Fig. 2**).[4] The high T2 signal intensity corresponds to areas of low attenuation on CT and reflects the high water content of the cartilaginous lesions.[1] The hypointense areas correspond to calcification on CT and radiographs and are more conspicuous on gradient echo images secondary to magnetic susceptibility effects.[1,4] The second most common pattern, seen in 14% of patients, lacked the focal areas of hypointensity because of lack of mineralization (**Fig. 3**).[4] The third pattern, seen in 9% of patients, demonstrated foci with central signal intensity isointense to fat with a peripheral low signal intensity rim, corresponding to foci of mature endochondral ossification.[4]

Pigmented villonodular synovitis

Pigmented villonodular synovitis (PVNS) is a benign proliferative synovial process that can occur in an intra-articular location or in a bursa or tendon sheath. The cause is debated; inflammatory processes, disorders of lipid metabolism, and recurrent intra-articular hemorrhage have all been proposed as potential causative factors.[5] However, given its association with characteristic cytogenetic abnormalities and potential for autonomous growth, some authors believe that it is a true neoplastic process.[5,6] A hallmark of this disorder is the absence of calcification, which is extremely rare in the setting of PVNS. In fact, the presence of calcification essentially excludes the diagnosis of PVNS and other entities, such as PSC and synovial sarcoma, should be considered. Malignant PVNS has been reported, but it is exceedingly rare and difficult to distinguish from benign disease unless there is extensive bone marrow invasion or distant metastatic disease.[5,7]

PVNS presents in two morphologically distinct forms: a diffuse form that involves an entire joint, and a focal nodular form that can be intra- or extra-articular (discussed later). The diffuse form of PVNS classically affects a single joint. The knee is the most common articulation affected, followed by the hip. The clinical presentation varies, but patients often present with pain, swelling, and/or limited range of motion, thus mimicking internal derangement of the knee. An associated

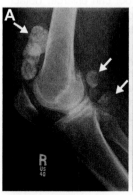
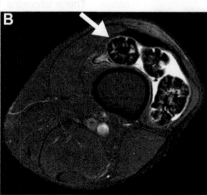

Fig. 1. (*A*) Lateral radiograph of the knee demonstrates several large ossified intra-articular bodies within the suprapatellar recess, posterior joint, and subpopliteal recess (*arrows*). The presence of underlying severe osteoarthrosis and the variable size and shape of the bodies is typical of secondary synovial osteochondromatosis. (*B*) Axial proton-density-weighted fat-suppressed image through the suprapatellar recess shows three large heterogenous intra-articular bodies (*arrow*) that are predominantly low signal intensity because of mineralization.

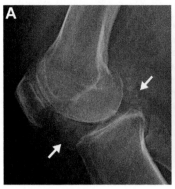
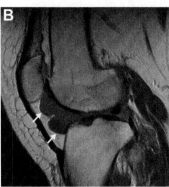

Fig. 2. (*A*) Lateral radiograph of the knee demonstrates a moderate joint effusion with clustered small foci of calcification/ossification, predominantly at the infrapatellar fat pad and posterior aspect of the joint (*arrows*). (*B*) Sagittal proton-density-weighted image demonstrates synovial hypertrophy eroding into the infrapatellar fat pad containing multiple small hypointense foci (*arrows*) corresponding to the calcifications seen on the radiographs. Focal involvement like this suggests early disease; typically the entire synovial lining is affected.

large joint effusion is common, particularly in large joints, such as the knee.[8] Erosion of the bone takes place in advanced disease, occurring most commonly in smaller joints with a tight capsule. Erosions are detected in 60% of cases at MR imaging versus 26% to 32% at radiography.[8] Total synovectomy is usually required and recurrence is common, typically managed with repeat surgery and/or adjuvant radiation therapy.[5]

When the diffuse form of PVNS affects the knee, radiographs typically show a large nonspecific effusion, relative joint space preservation, and a lack of erosions unless the disease is particularly severe and long-standing. MR imaging is the imaging modality of choice, showing diffuse, plaque-like synovial thickening throughout the joint with nodularity of the abnormal synovium.[5,8] A villous or villonodular morphology of the diseased synovium can also be seen but is less common.[5] Unlike most synovial disorders, the synovial proliferation demonstrates low to intermediate signal intensity on T1- and T2-weighted sequences with scattered deposition of hemosiderin throughout the joint. The hemosiderin accounts for the characteristic

low T2 signal intensity and increased prominence of these low signal intensity areas ("blooming") on gradient echo images (**Fig. 4**).[5] Although hemosiderin deposition can also occur in the setting of synovial hemangioma and hemophilic arthropathy, PVNS is distinguished from these entities by the absence of serpentine vascular channels typical of synovial hemangioma and the lack of a clinical history of hemophilia.[5] Postcontrast enhancement is a common feature but the degree of enhancement is variable.[5,9]

Lipoma arborescens

Lipoma arborescens is an uncommon benign villous lipomatous proliferation of the synovial membrane.[10,11] It is not a true neoplasm and most commonly develops as a secondary reactive process in a joint affected by chronic inflammatory synovitis or osteoarthrosis.[12] Far less commonly, a primary form of lipoma arborescens can develop in a joint with no underlying pathologic process.[10] Lipoma arborescens is usually monoarticular and most commonly occurs in the suprapatellar recess of the knee, although it can affect any joint and has

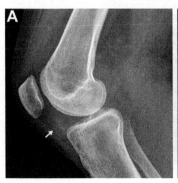
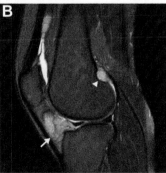

Fig. 3. (*A*) Lateral radiograph of the knee demonstrates a small joint effusion and soft tissue effacement of the infrapatellar fat pad (*arrow*). No calcifications are present. (*B*) Sagittal T2-weighted fat-suppressed images demonstrate extensive lobulated intra-articular T2-hyperintense signal intensity with extension into the infrapatellar fat pad (*arrow*). Note that there is posterior involvement as well, with resultant early erosion of the posterior femoral cortex (*arrowhead*). Pathology demonstrated synovial chondromatosis, presumably early in the disease course because it had not yet ossified.

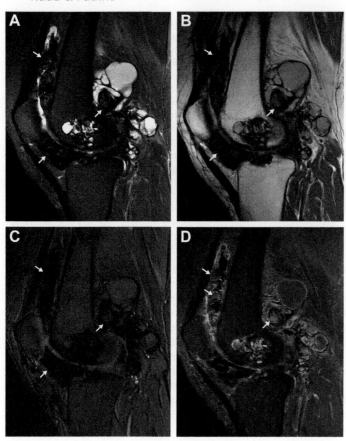

Fig. 4. Sagittal T2-weighted fat-suppressed (A), proton-density-weighted (B), and gradient echo images (C) demonstrate extensive intra-articular low-signal intensity tissue throughout the knee with "blooming" on the gradient echo image (arrows). Sagittal T1-weighted fat-suppressed postcontrast image (D) demonstrates heterogeneous enhancement (arrows).

also been reported within bursae.[10,11] It is typically diagnosed in the fifth to seventh decade of life and patients most often present with slowly progressive painless swelling and recurrent joint effusions.[13] Conservative management is typically implemented. In advanced symptomatic cases, a synovectomy is performed with little risk of recurrence.

Radiography can show a large effusion and in rare cases, the fatty proliferation may be evident. However, MR imaging is far more accurate, demonstrating villous or frondlike adipose proliferation of the subsynovial tissue with signal intensity following fat on all sequences (**Fig. 5**).[11,14] On postcontrast images, there is no enhancement of the adipose proliferation, although there can be enhancement of the underlying synovium if it is inflamed. A joint effusion is almost always present. Osseous erosions have been described. However, they are typically seen in small tight joints rather than at the knee joint, which is more capacious and less prone to mass affect and bone erosion.[11,15]

Focal Neoplasms and Nonneoplastic Masses

Localized nodular synovitis
Localized nodular synovitis is the focal masslike form of PVNS that most frequently develops within the tendon sheaths of the hands and feet. Less frequently, it develops within a joint, most commonly within the infrapatellar fat pad of the knee.[16] Although it shares similar histologic features with PVNS, it involves a smaller region of synovium, has less hemosiderin deposition, lacks a hemorrhagic joint effusion, and has a smooth surface rather than plaquelike thickening with nodularity.[16] Treatment consists of local excision and recurrence is uncommon.

There is nothing specific about the mass on radiography or CT and the MR imaging appearance of intra-articular localized nodular synovitis is more variable than in the diffuse form of PVNS. The mass can appear as a small, well-circumscribed ovoid lesion or a larger multilobulated lesion. It is typically isointense or hyperintense to muscle on T1-weighted images and variable in signal intensity on T2-weighted images.[16] Enhancement is seen on postcontrast images because of the presence of capillary proliferation in these lesions (**Fig. 6**).[17] Intermixed hypointense areas may be seen and represent regions of high hemosiderin concentration, which demonstrates increased conspicuity on gradient echo images.[16] A central cleftlike or linear hyperintense region on T2-weighted images has been described in some cases, which may represent necrosis or entrapped joint fluid.[5,16]

Cyclops lesion

The cyclops lesion is not a true neoplasm. Rather, it is a reactive nodular mass of fibrous granulation tissue that forms in the anterior intercondylar notch typically adjacent to an anterior cruciate ligament (ACL) graft. However, similar lesions have been reported following ligament injury in the absence of surgical reconstruction.[18,19] In the postoperative setting, it has been suggested that the tissue proliferation is a reaction to debris from drilling of the tibial tunnel or an inflammatory response to repetitive microtrauma of the graft.[20] Two distinct histologic subtypes have been described, the true cyclops lesion and a "cyclopoid" lesion, although these are indistinguishable on MR imaging.[21] The true cyclops lesion is composed of fibrocartilaginous tissue with active central bone formation making it harder and more likely to produce symptoms, whereas the "cyclopoid" lesion is composed of fibrocartilaginous tissue with surrounding granulation tissue.[21]

The "cyclops syndrome" is a clinical diagnosis that is made when the mass acts as a mechanical obstruction, which limits full knee extension and produces an audible and palpable "clunk" at terminal extension.[22] Although symptomatic lesions require arthroscopic debridement, the advent of MR imaging has shown that cyclops lesions are common following ACL surgery and that most are asymptomatic and can be managed conservatively. A prospective study by Facchetti and colleagues[20] found that cyclops lesions are detected on MR imaging at 6 months postoperatively in 25% of patients, and that neither the presence nor the size of the lesion within the first 2 years after surgery is associated with inferior clinical outcome.

MR imaging has high (>85%) sensitivity, specificity, and accuracy for the detection of postoperative cyclops lesions.[18] They appear as well-circumscribed, sessile or pedunculated nodules located anterior to the ACL graft, with a mean size of 13 × 12 × 12 mm.[18] They are typically hypointense to intermediate on T1-weighted images and exhibit variable, more heterogeneous signal on fluid-sensitive sequences (**Fig. 7**).[20] Areas of ossification may be seen within the mass, appearing as irregular circumscribed foci with fat signal on all pulse sequences. In the absence of internal ossification or a history of ACL surgery, the mass is difficult to distinguish from localized nodular synovitis, which has overlapping imaging and histologic features. The most useful imaging feature differentiating a cyclops lesion from focal nodular synovitis is its more intimate association with the ACL or ACL remnant.[19]

Synovial lipoma

Focal intra-articular synovial lipoma is far less common than diffuse lipoma arborescens as a cause for a fat signal mass within the joint. A recent review by Poorteman and colleagues[23] identified only 21 reported cases of true synovial lipoma, 18 of which occurred in the knee. It typically arises de novo, unrelated to other joint pathology. This is in contrast to lipoma arborescens, which is usually a secondary reactive process to chronic inflammatory synovitis or osteoarthrosis.[24] Synovial lipomas typically present as well-circumscribed lesions with a thin fibrous capsule and a vascular pedicle demonstrating signal isointense to fat on all MR imaging sequences. Occasionally, osseous metaplasia may occur and areas of calcification or ossification may be seen within the lesion (**Fig. 8**).[24,25] The cause of the osseous metaplasia is unclear. Some authors speculate that prior trauma may be the inciting event.[24] However, there are case reports of osseous metaplasia in the absence of prior trauma. These lesions can cause locking by impinging on the articular surfaces, intercondylar

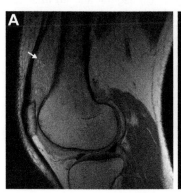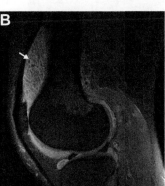

Fig. 5. Sagittal proton-density-weighted (*A*) and short tau inversion recovery (*B*) images demonstrate frondlike adipose proliferation of the subsynovial tissue in the suprapatellar recess (*arrows*) with an associated large joint effusion.

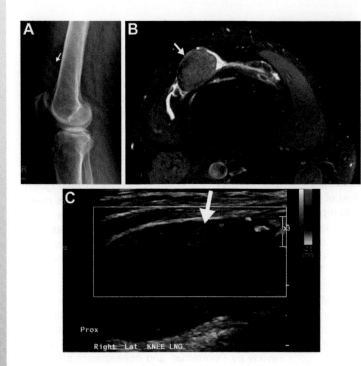

Fig. 6. (*A*) Lateral radiograph demonstrates an ovoid soft tissue mass projecting over the suprapatellar recess (*arrow*). (*B*) Axial proton-density-weighted fat-suppressed image demonstrates a well-circumscribed mass in the suprapatellar recess (*arrow*). The mass is slightly hyperintense to skeletal muscle with a few intermixed areas of low signal intensity. Given that the MR imaging features lacked specificity, ultrasound-guided biopsy was recommended. (*C*) Ultrasound demonstrated a heterogeneous hypoechoic mass with mild internal vascularity (*arrow*). Pathology was consistent with localized nodular synovitis. (*Courtesy of* Karen Chen, MD, San Diego VA Medical Center San Diego, California.)

notch, or the menisci.[23] Patients may also present with acute pain if there is torsion of the vascular pedicle.[26] Treatment of symptomatic lesions consists of surgical resection.

Synovial hemangioma

Synovial hemangiomas are rare benign vascular lesions that typically occur in children and young adults, with approximately 75% of cases presenting before the age of 16.[27] Histologically, they are classified similar to other soft tissue hemangiomas into cavernous, capillary, arteriovenous, and venous subtypes, with the cavernous subtype being the most common pattern seen.[28,29] Hemangiomas that occur within or near a joint can also be

subclassified as intra-articular, juxta-articular, and intermediate (intra- and extra-articular components).[28] The term synovial hemangioma should be reserved for the intra-articular and intermediate subtypes.[28] They predominantly occur in the knee, but have also been reported in the elbow, wrist, ankle, and temporomandibular joints.[28–30] Symptoms are nonspecific and include pain, swelling, limited range of motion, and spontaneous hemarthrosis, often resulting in delayed diagnosis and the risk of articular damage secondary to recurrent hemarthrosis.[14,28] Early surgical excision is used to prevent irreversible arthropathy using arthroscopic resection for well-circumscribed or pedunculated lesions and open excision for

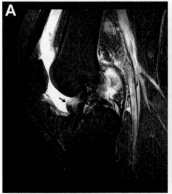
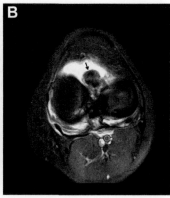

Fig. 7. (*A*) Sagittal and (*B*) axial T2-weighted fat-suppressed images demonstrate a well-circumscribed heterogeneously hypointense nodule in the anterior intercondylar notch adjacent to the ACL graft (*arrows*).

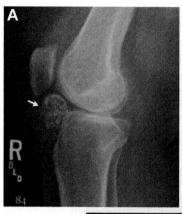
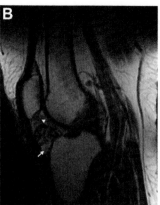

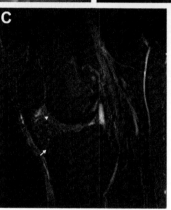

Fig. 8. (*A*) Lateral radiograph of the knee demonstrates a calcified mass centered in the infrapatellar fat pad (*arrow*). Sagittal T1-weighted (*B*) and T2-weighted fat-suppressed (*C*) images demonstrate that the mass is primarily composed of macroscopic fat (*arrows*) with additional internal hypointense foci (*arrowheads*) corresponding to the calcifications seen on the radiograph.

lesions that are diffuse.[28,31] Recurrence is common in diffuse lesions because they typically infiltrate adjacent structures, making it challenging to achieve negative surgical margins.[32] Minimally invasive therapies, such as ethanol sclerotherapy, have been shown to be efficacious in palliating pain and reducing lesion size but are rarely curative.[32]

Radiographs are normal in more than half of patients but may demonstrate a nonspecific soft tissue mass about the joint, joint effusion, decreased bone mineralization, or advanced maturation of the epiphysis. The identification of multiple phleboliths adds considerable specificity. Arthropathy simulating hemophilic arthritis may be seen in patients with recurrent hemarthrosis from these lesions.[28] Ultrasound can also be used for lesion characterization, especially in young patients who would require sedation for the MR imaging and for serial follow-up of lesions. The sonographic features are similar to other soft tissue hemangiomas of the extremities and includes a complex mass with shadowing echogenic foci if phleboliths are present. At Doppler evaluation, there may be low-resistance arterial flow with forward flow during systole and diastole.[33]

The MR imaging features are often pathognomonic. Findings include a lobulated mass arising from the synovium that is purely intra-articular or has intra-articular and extra-articular components. They are intermediate in signal intensity on T1-weighted images and markedly hyperintense on T2-weighted images, which likely reflects pooling of blood within vascular spaces.[14] Linear T2 hypointense intralesional septations, fluid-fluid levels, and hemosiderin deposition are also commonly seen (**Fig. 9**).[28,29] The presence of serpentine vascular channels and phleboliths within the vascular spaces allows specific diagnosis and distinguishes hemangioma from PVNS, which can also have considerable hemosiderin deposition.[5] MR angiography can also be performed for dynamic assessment and better characterization of the vascular anatomy for preoperative planning. Given its exquisite temporal resolution, MR angiography allows differentiation of synovial hemangiomas from high-flow vascular malformations, such as arteriovenous malformations, which typically demonstrate a central nidus of tangled vessels and enlarged rapidly draining veins.[28]

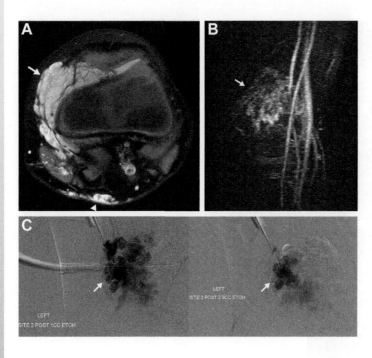

Fig. 9. (A) Axial proton-density-weighted fat-suppressed image demonstrates a lobulated markedly hyperintense mass with serpentine morphology and thin hypointense intralesional septations (*arrow*). The epicenter of the mass is extra-articular at the medial aspect of the knee, but there is intracapsular extension through the medial patellar retinaculum to involve the prefemoral fat pad. There is an additional extra-articular component, which involves the posterior subcutaneous soft tissues (*arrowhead*). (B) Maximum intensity projection image from an MR angiographic examination in the venous phase shows pooling of contrast in the hemangioma (*arrow*), which demonstrated slow filling and absence of an early draining vein on dynamic imaging, consistent with a low-flow vascular lesion. (C) Digital subtraction angiography status post-injection of 1 mL and 2.5 mL of ethanol demonstrates progressive decrease in opacification of the lesion (*arrows*).

Intra-articular ganglion cyst

A ganglion cyst is a tumorlike well-marginated mass filled with gelatinous fluid and surrounded by a dense connective tissue capsule.[34,35] The pathogenesis of ganglion cyst formation is unclear, but it is hypothesized that they result either from mucinous degeneration of connective tissues or herniation of synovial tissue through a defect in the joint capsule or tendon sheath.[35,36] Although there is no universally accepted classification system for ganglion cysts, it is useful to categorize them based on location into juxta-articular, intra-articular, and periosteal categories, with the juxta-articular type being the most common form.[35] At the knee joint, the reported prevalence of intra-articular ganglion cysts at MR imaging of the knee is approximately 1%.[37–39] Most arise within or adjacent to the cruciate ligaments, with the tibial insertion of the ACL being the most common location.[37,38] Although pericruciate ganglion cysts and mucoid degeneration of the underlying cruciate ligament often coexist, the precise relationship between these two entities remains unclear because cysts can develop near a normal-appearing ACL.[38] They have also been described arising in the infrapatellar fat pad or from the posterior joint capsule.[35,37]

Most ganglion cysts are asymptomatic and discovered incidentally; those that are symptomatic tend to be larger and intimate with the cruciate ligaments where they can interfere with normal knee motion. Cysts anterior to the ACL typically limit extension, whereas those posterior to the cruciate ligaments limit flexion.[40] Although asymptomatic ganglion cysts are managed conservatively, treatment considerations for symptomatic lesions include excision, percutaneous aspiration, and intralesional corticosteroid injection.

The MR imaging appearance of a ganglion cyst is characteristic. The cyst appears as a well-defined, unilocular or multilocular mass, with or without septations, with signal intensity similar to that of fluid on all pulse sequences (**Fig. 10**).[41] The signal intensity is typically homogeneous, but in long-standing lesions, especially those complicated by prior hemorrhage or infection, the signal may be more complex. A low signal intensity peripheral rim may be seen, corresponding to a fibrous capsule.[41] Postcontrast imaging is especially useful for distinguishing a ganglion from solid lesions that can have overlapping features on conventional MR imaging sequences. Following intravenous contrast enhancement, ganglion cysts classically demonstrate a thin peripheral rim of enhancement with no enhancement of the central fluid component. Central nodular or diffuse enhancement indicates the mass has solid elements and excludes ganglion cyst from the differential diagnosis.

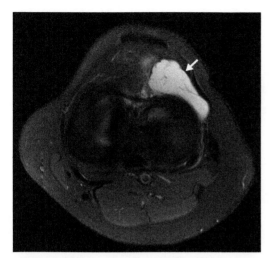

Fig. 10. Axial proton-density fat-suppressed image demonstrates a multiloculated cystic mass with thin internal septations within the infrapatellar fat pad anterior to the lateral meniscus (*arrow*). The lesion was symptomatic and went on to surgical resection. Pathology confirmed a benign ganglion cyst. The lateral meniscus was intact at arthroscopy.

Synovial sarcoma

Synovial sarcomas account for 3% to 11% of all primary malignant soft tissue neoplasms.[42] They typically present in adolescents and young adults at a mean age of 32 years.[43] The name is a misnomer, because these tumors do not arise from synovium but rather are thought to originate from primitive mesenchymal cells that differentiate into cells that appear similar histologically to synovial cells.[43] Approximately 95% occur in the extremities. Most are periarticular, developing within 5 cm of a joint, with the popliteal fossa being the most common site.[42,44–46] Although popliteal synovial sarcoma can invade the knee joint, typically through a defect in the posterior joint capsule,[42] they originate outside the articulation. Only 5% to 10% of synovial sarcomas actually form within an articulation, most commonly at the anterior knee within the infrapatellar fat pad.[42] Synovial sarcomas are intermediate- to high-grade malignancies. Wide local excision is the treatment of choice for localized disease. The role of adjuvant therapy remains controversial.[42] Unfortunately, local recurrence and metastasis is common and prognosis is guarded.

Conventional radiology has poor sensitivity for detection unless the mass is large and calcified, which occurs in 30% of cases as fine stippled calcifications dispersed within the lesion, best appreciated with CT.[42] MR imaging is the modality of choice for assessment, although calcification often appears less extensive.[42] On MR imaging, the lesion

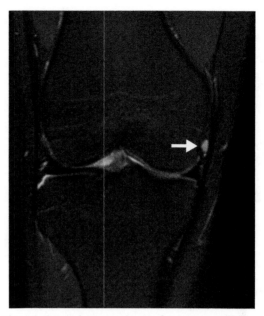

Fig. 11. Coronal proton-density fat-suppressed image demonstrates a small hyperintense nodule deep to the superficial medial collateral ligament at the level of the medial femoral condyle. The lesion was palpable and tender, so the patient went on to surgical resection and pathology revealed biphasic-type synovial sarcoma.

is typically nonspecific in appearance, isointense to slightly hyperintense to skeletal muscle on T1-weighted and hyperintense on T2-weighted images with a heterogenous multilobulated appearance. Synovial sarcomas typically arise in an intermuscular location, resulting in the "split-fat" sign, although invasion into surrounding muscles is common. Osseous invasion is seen in 21% of cases and neurovascular encasement is seen in 17% to 24% of cases.[42,45,47] Postcontrast images demonstrate heterogeneous enhancement in 83% to 100% of lesions.[42,45] The "triple sign" refers to the simultaneous appearance of regions of low, intermediate, and high signal intensity on T2-weighted images within the mass.[45] This represents the admixture of solid cellular elements (intermediate signal intensity), hemorrhage or necrosis (high signal intensity), and calcified or fibrotic collagenized tissue (low signal intensity).[42] A "bowl of grapes" appearance has also been described, characterized by large cystic areas, foci of hemorrhage, and fluid levels.[42] These signs lack specificity because they are found in a range of malignancies. In addition, there is a wide range of MR imaging appearances in synovial sarcoma, including small size, smooth contour, homogeneous signal, and lack of invasion into adjacent structures that can simulate the appearance of a nonaggressive lesion (**Fig. 11**).[43,48]

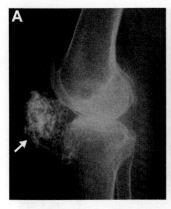
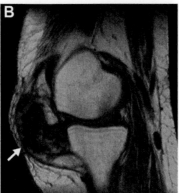

Fig. 12. (*A*) Lateral radiograph of the knee demonstrates a large partially calcified mass centered within the infrapatellar fat pad (*arrow*). The adjacent bone appears normal. (*B*) Sagittal T1-weighted image demonstrates that the mass is heterogeneous but predominantly hypointense (*arrow*) because of the calcifications. (*Courtesy of* Dexter Witte, MD, Baptist Hospital, Memphis, Tenn.)

Extraskeletal chondroma

Extraskeletal chondroma is a rare benign tumor that can form within (intra-articular chondroma) or adjacent (para-articular chondroma) to the joint. They occur most commonly at the knee, although other joints, such as the hip and elbow, may be affected.[49] The mass is thought to arise from cartilaginous metaplasia of the joint capsule or its adjacent connective tissue, forming a cartilaginous mass most commonly seen within Hoffa's fat pad at the anterior knee.[49,50] The mass develops variable degrees of ossification as it matures, producing small flecks of mineralization or large bizarre areas of ossification that are most apparent on radiographs or CT. This entity, although rare, should be considered in the differential diagnosis of a mineralized articular mass. Unlike primary synovial osteochondromatosis, the mineralization of intra-articular chondroma is focal, typically limited to the infrapatellar fat pad, and generally more bizarre and confluent.[50] Differentiation of a para-articular chondroma from fat necrosis, a calcified synovial sarcoma, or an ossified lipoma is difficult based on the imaging appearance alone and tissue sampling may be required.[51]

Although CT is preferred for visualizing mineralization within the mass, MR imaging has also been used for diagnosis, classically demonstrating a large round or lobulated mass centered within the infrapatellar fat pad. The tumor is typically large when diagnosed, ranging in size from 2.2 to 10 cm, and may be associated with erosion of the adjacent anterosuperior tibia.[50] The mass is predominantly isointense to hypointense to skeletal muscle on T1-weighted images. However, in cases where ossification is present, areas of T1 hyperintensity are seen. On T2-weighted images, the masses are heterogeneously hyperintense, with the hyperintense areas corresponding to the

hyaline cartilaginous tissue (**Fig. 12**).[50] Postcontrast images may demonstrate peripheral enhancement of the cartilage lobules. Surgical excision is the treatment of choice and local recurrence is rare.[50]

CLINICS CARE POINTS

- The MR imaging of primary synovial chondromatosis varies depending on whether mineralization is absent or present and on the maturity of that mineralization. The disorder is initially nonmineralized, then develops faint chondroid calcifications and ultimately contains mature endochondral ossification.

- Hemosiderin deposition and the absence of mineralization are the imaging hallmarks of diffuse PVNS. The hemosiderin deposition results in its characteristic low T2 signal with blooming on gradient echo imaging. Localized nodular synovitis shares similar histologic features but shows focal disease with less hemosiderin deposition.

- Tumors and tumor-like diseases within joints can result in extrinsic erosion of bone secondary to mass effect causing chronic pressure. This type of erosion is most common in small joints with tight capsules and occurs less commonly at the knee due to its large capacious capsule.

DISCLOSURE

The authors have nothing to disclose.

REFERENCES

1. Murphey MD, Vidal JA, Fanburg-Smith JC, et al. Imaging of synovial chondromatosis with radiologic-

pathologic correlation. Radiographics 2007;27(5): 1465–88.

2. McCarthy C, Anderson WJ, Vlychou M, et al. Primary synovial chondromatosis: a reassessment of malignant potential in 155 cases. Skeletal Radiol 2016; 45(6):755–62.

3. Wittkop B, Davies AM, Mangham DC. Primary synovial chondromatosis and synovial chondrosarcoma: a pictorial review. Eur Radiol 2002;12(8):2112–9.

4. Kramer J, Recht M, Deely DM, et al. MR appearance of idiopathic synovial osteochondromatosis. J Comput Assist Tomogr 1993;17(5):772–6.

5. Murphey MD, Rhee JH, Lewis RB, et al. Pigmented villonodular synovitis: radiologic-pathologic correlation. Radiographics 2008;28(5):1493–518.

6. Temponi EF, Barros AAG, Paganini VO, et al. Diffuse pigmented villonodular synovitis in knee joint: diagnosis and treatment. Rev Bras Ortop 2017;52(4): 450–7.

7. Kalil RK, Unni KK. Malignancy in pigmented villonodular synovitis. Skeletal Radiol 1998;27:392–5.

8. Hughes TH, Sartoris DJ, Schweitzer ME, et al. Pigmented villonodular synovitis: MRI characteristics. Skeletal Radiol 1995;24:7–12.

9. Lin J, Jacobson JA, Jamadar DA, et al. Pigmented villonodular synovitis and related lesions: the spectrum of imaging findings. AJR Am J Roentgenol 1999;172:191–7.

10. Vilanova JC, Barceló J, Villalón M, et al. MR imaging of lipoma arborescens and the associated lesions. Skeletal Radiol 2003;32(9):504–9.

11. Ryu KN, Jaovisidha S, Schweitzer M, et al. MR imaging of lipoma arborescens of the knee joint. AJR Am J Roentgenol 1996;167(5):1229–32.

12. Hallel T, Lew S, Bansal M. Villous lipomatous proliferation of the synovial membrane (lipoma arborescens). J Bone Joint Surg Am 1988;70(2):264–70.

13. Martin S, Hernandez L, Romero J, et al. Diagnostic imaging of lipoma arborescens. Skeletal Radiol 1998;27:325–9.

14. Sheldon PJ, Forrester DM, Learch TJ. Imaging of intra-articular masses. Radiographics 2005;25(1):105–19.

15. Chae EY, Chung HW, Shin MJ, et al. Lipoma arborescens of the glenohumeral joint causing bone erosion: MRI features with gadolinium enhancement. Skeletal Radiol 2009;38(8):815–8.

16. Huang GS, Lee CH, Chan WP, et al. Localized nodular synovitis of the knee: MR imaging appearance and clinical correlates in 21 patients. AJR Am J Roentgenol 2003;181(2):539–43.

17. De Beuckeleer L, De Schepper A, De Belder F, et al. Magnetic resonance imaging of localized giant cell tumour of the tendon sheath. Eur Radiol 1997;7: 198–201.

18. Bradley DM, Bergman AG, Dillingham MF. MR imaging of cyclops lesions. AJR Am J Roentgenol 2000; 174(3):719–26.

19. Runyan BR, Bancroft LW, Peterson JJ, et al. Cyclops lesions that occur in the absence of prior anterior ligament reconstruction. Radiographics 2007;27(6):e26.

20. Facchetti L, Schwaiger BJ, Gersing AS, et al. Cyclops lesions detected by MRI are frequent findings after ACL surgical reconstruction but do not impact clinical outcome over 2 years. Eur Radiol 2017;27(8):3499–508.

21. Muellner T, Kdolsky R, Großschmidt K, et al. Cyclops and cyclopoid formation after anterior cruciate ligament reconstruction: clinical and histomorphological differences. Knee Surg Sport Traumatol Arthrosc 1999;7(5):284–9.

22. Jackson DW, Schaefer RK. Cyclops syndrome: loss of extension following intra-articular anterior cruciate ligament reconstruction. Arthroscopy 1990;6:171–8.

23. Poorteman L, Declercq H, Natens P, et al. Intra-articular synovial lipoma of the knee joint. BJR Case Rep 2015;1(2):20150061.

24. Pudlowski R, Gilula L, Kyriakos M. Intraarticular lipoma with osseous metaplasia: radiographic-pathologic correlation. AJR Am J Roentgenol 1979; 132(3):471–3.

25. Huynh T-PV, Cipriano CA, Hagemann IS, et al. Osteolipoma of the knee. Radiol Case Rep 2017; 12(1):124–9.

26. Hirano K, Deguchi M, Kanamono T. Intra-articular synovial lipoma of the knee joint (located in the lateral recess): a case report and review of the literature. The Knee 2007;14:63–7.

27. Moon NF. Synovial hemangioma of the knee joint. A review of previously reported cases and inclusion of two new cases. Clin Orthop Relat Res 1973;90: 183–90.

28. Wen DW, Tan TJ, Rasheed S. Synovial haemangioma of the knee joint: an unusual cause of knee pain in a 14-month old girl. Skeletal Radiol 2016;45(6):827–31.

29. Greenspan A, Azouz EM, Matthews J 2nd, et al. Synovial hemangioma: imaging features in eight histologically proven cases, review of the literature, and differential diagnosis. Skeletal Radiol 1995;24(8): 583–90.

30. Devaney K, Vinh TN, Sweet DE. Synovial hemangioma: a report of 20 cases with differential diagnostic considerations. Hum Pathol 1993;24(7):737–45.

31. Price NJ, Cundy PJ. Synovial hemangioma of the knee. J Pediatr Orthop 1997;17(1):74–7.

32. Crawford EA, Slotcavage RL, King JJ, et al. Ethanol sclerotherapy reduces pain in symptomatic musculoskeletal hemangiomas. Clin Orthop Relat Res 2009;467(11):2955–61.

33. Olsen KI, Stacy GS, Montag A. Soft-tissue cavernous hemangioma. Radiographics 2004;24(3):849–54.

34. Perdikakis E, Skiadas V. MRI characteristics of cysts and "cyst-like" lesions in and around the knee: what the radiologist needs to know. Insights Imaging 2013;4(3):257–72.

35. Beaman FD, Peterson JJ. MR imaging of cysts, ganglia, and bursae about the knee. Magn Reson Imaging Clin North Am 2007;15(1):39–52.

36. Angelides AC, Wallace PF. The dorsal ganglion of the wrist: its pathogenesis, gross microscopic anatomy and surgical treatment. J Hand Surg Am 1976; 1:228–35.

37. Bui-Mansfield LT, Youngberg RA. Intraarticular ganglia of the knee: prevalence, presentation, etiology, and management. AJR Am J Roentgenol 1997; 168:123–7.

38. Bergin D, Morrison WB, Carrino JA, et al. Anterior cruciate ligament ganglia and mucoid degeneration: coexistence and clinical correlation. AJR Am J Roentgenol 2004;182:1283–7.

39. Kim MG, Kim BH, Choi JA, et al. Intra-articular ganglion cysts of the knee: clinical and MR imaging features. Eur Radiol 2001;11:834–40.

40. Krudwig WK, Schulte KK, Heinemann C. Intra-articular ganglion cysts of the knee joint: a report of 85 cases and review of the literature. Knee Surgery, Sports Traumatol Arthrosc 2004;12:123–9.

41. Steinbach LS, Stevens KJ. Imaging of cysts and bursae about the knee. Radiol Clin North Am 2013; 51(3):433–54.

42. Murphey MD, Gibson MS, Jennings BT, et al. From the archives of the AFIP: Imaging of synovial sarcoma with radiologic-pathologic correlation. Radiographics 2006;26(5):1543–65.

43. Bakri A, Shinagare AB, Krajewski KM, et al. Synovial sarcoma: imaging features of common and uncommon primary sites, metastatic patterns, and treatment response. AJR Am J Roentgenol 2012; 199(2):W208–15.

44. Spillane AJ, A'Hern R, Judson IR, et al. Synovial sarcoma: a clinicopathologic, staging, and prognostic assessment. J Clin Oncol 2000;18(22):3794–803.

45. Jones BC, Sundaram M, Kransdorf MJ. Synovial sarcoma: MR imaging findings in 34 patients. AJR Am J Roentgenol 1993;161(4):827–30.

46. Shah A, James SL, Davies AM, et al. A diagnostic approach to popliteal fossa masses. Clin Radiol 2017;72(4):323–37.

47. Horowitz AL, Resnick D, Watson RC. The roentgen features of synovial sarcomas. Clin Radiol 1973; 24(4):481–4.

48. Blacksin MF, Siegel JR, Benevenia J, et al. Synovial sarcoma: frequency of nonaggressive MR characteristics. J Comput Assist Tomogr 1997;21(5):785–9.

49. Helpert C, Davies AM, Evans N, et al. Differential diagnosis of tumours and tumour-like lesions of the infrapatellar (Hoffa's) fat pad: pictorial review with an emphasis on MR imaging. Eur Radiol 2004; 14(12):2337–46.

50. González-Lois C, García-de-la-Torre P, Santos Briz-Terrón A, et al. Intracapsular and para-articular chondroma adjacent to large joints: report of three cases and review of the literature. Skeletal Radiol 2001;30(12):672–6.

51. Stacy GS, Heck RK, Peabody TD, et al. Neoplastic and tumorlike lesions detected on MR imaging of the knee in patients with suspected internal derangement: Part 2, articular and juxtaarticular entities. AJR Am J Roentgenol 2002;178(3):595–9.

MR Imaging of the Postoperative Meniscus

Sonja Fierstra, MD[a], Lawrence M. White, MD, FRCPC[a,b,*]

KEYWORDS

- Magnetic resonance imaging • Meniscus • Meniscal tear • Meniscectomy • Meniscal repair
- Posterior meniscus root repair • Postoperative imaging

KEY POINTS

- Surfacing high T2-weighted "fluid" signal, abnormal meniscal morphology, and displaced meniscal tissue are MR imaging criteria for a meniscal retear.
- The accuracy of conventional MR imaging and MR arthrography (MRA) for the detection of a retear is equivalent after low-grade partial meniscal excision (<25%).
- Following higher-grade meniscectomies (>25%) and meniscal repair, MRA and computed tomographic arthrography can be helpful adjunct diagnostic techniques.

INTRODUCTION

Meniscal tears are one of the most common knee injuries sustained, and meniscal surgery is one of the most frequent orthopedic procedures, with approximately one million meniscal surgeries performed in the United States per year.[1]

Following arthroscopic treatment of a torn meniscus, a recurrent or residual meniscal tear may present with clinical symptoms of new knee swelling, pain, or mechanical derangement in the treated knee. If findings on physical examination are suggestive of possible recurrent meniscal pathologic condition and radiographs exclude the presence of an acute fracture or advanced osteoarthritis, advanced imaging may be indicated in the evaluation of the postoperative meniscus and the knee joint.

MR imaging performed without or with intraarticular contrast agent is currently the examination of choice for assessing patients who have recurrent symptoms after meniscus surgery. However, the evaluation of the postoperative meniscus with MR imaging can be challenging, as expected postoperative changes in the setting of an intact uncomplicated postoperative meniscus can demonstrate features relied on to diagnose a meniscal tear in the nonoperative knee.

NORMAL ANATOMY

The function of the menisci is primarily to distribute weight-bearing forces at the knee and protect hyaline articular cartilage, while contributing to knee stability and likely proprioception and cartilage nourishment.[2] Collagen bundles are primarily responsible for the tensile strength of menisci, with longitudinal circumferential orientation of meniscal collagen bundles functioning to transfer vertical compressive load into circumferential "hoop stress." The outer vascularized one-third of the meniscus is referred to as the red zone because of its blood supply facilitating meniscal healing. In contrast, the inner one-third of the meniscus, known as white zone, is considered avascular, with associated limited intrinsic healing capacity.[3]

Anatomically, the menisci are divided into 3 portions, consisting of the anterior horn, meniscal body, and posterior horn. The medial meniscus has a more open C-shape configuration, while the lateral meniscus is more rounded with a closed

[a] Joint Department of Medical Imaging, University Health Network, Mount Sinai Hospital and Women's College Hospital, 600 University Avenue, Toronto, Ontario M5G 1X5 Canada; [b] Department of Medical Imaging, Temerty Faculty of Medicine, University of Toronto, Toronto, Ontario, Canada
* Corresponding author. Joint Department of Medical Imaging, University Health Network, Mount Sinai Hospital and Women's College Hospital, 600 University Avenue, Toronto, Ontario M5G 1X5 Canada.
E-mail address: Lawrence.white@uhn.ca

Magn Reson Imaging Clin N Am 30 (2022) 351–362
https://doi.org/10.1016/j.mric.2021.11.012

C-shape morphology. The medial meniscus gradually increases in width from anterior to posterior, with its posterior horn being larger than the anterior horn. The lateral meniscus, in contrast, maintains a relatively constant width with anterior and posterior horns being similar in size.[4] The medial meniscus is more vulnerable to injury than the lateral meniscus because of its intimate attachment to the medial collateral ligament and tight meniscotibial ligamentous attachments (coronary ligament). In contrast, the lateral meniscus is more mobile and less prone to tearing except in the setting of anterior cruciate ligament (ACL) injury, where an increased relative incidence of lateral meniscal tears is observed.

The normal meniscus appears hypointense on T1- and T2-weighted MR images because of their fibrocartilaginous composition with high intrameniscal collagen content.[5] The C-shape configuration of the meniscus is well demonstrated on axial images. On coronal images, the meniscal body is seen as a triangular or wedge-shaped structure with its inner/apical free edge pointing to the intercondylar notch. On sagittal images, the anterior and posterior horns have a wedge-shaped configuration, whereas the meniscal body takes on a more "bow-tie" configuration.[6]

MENISCAL TEAR TREATMENT

Arthroscopic partial meniscectomy and meniscal repair are the main surgical considerations for treatment of meniscal tears. Posterior meniscus root repair is a newer arthroscopic repair technique. The primary aim of any meniscal surgery is to reestablish stability of the residual meniscus and preserve as much stable and viable meniscal tissue as possible.[7] The importance of maintaining meniscal tissue is a direct reflection of the understanding and recognition of meniscal insufficiency as a primary risk factor in the development and progression of articular cartilage damage and knee joint osteoarthritis.

Partial Meniscectomy

The goal of partial meniscectomy is to remove any unstable or displaced meniscal tissue and surgically trim the meniscus, leaving behind stable tissue capable of providing continued cushioning effects for the knee. Typically, partial meniscectomies are performed for tears involving the avascular white zone of the meniscus, which is considered to have limited primary healing capacity. Radial apical tears, displaced flap tears, and horizontal cleavage tears are generally considered not amenable for surgical repair and thus are commonly treated with partial meniscectomy.[8]

Meniscus Repair

As the primary principle of meniscal surgery is preservation of as much native stable meniscal tissue as feasible, the emphasis of modern surgical techniques has been focused on meniscal repair rather than meniscectomy whenever possible. Meniscal repairs are typically performed in management of tears involving the vascular red zone of the meniscus. Additional features that have been shown to be associated with improved meniscal healing following repair include tear location involving the lateral rather than medial meniscus, tear length of less than 25 mm, acute rather than chronic nature of the tear, patient age less than 30 years, and ligamentous stability of the joint.[9]

Posterior Meniscus Root Repair

Avulsion injuries or radial tears of the meniscus adjacent to its anterior or posterior attachment sites to the tibia are defined as meniscal root tears.[10] The posterior meniscus root insertion is an important and common site of meniscal root tearing. Lateral meniscus posterior root tears are usually seen associated with acute tears of the ACL, whereas medial meniscal posterior root tears are mainly the result of degenerative meniscal tearing.[11]

Posterior meniscal root tears can lead to meniscal extrusion from the joint line, loss of meniscal hoop tension, loss of load-bearing ability, and increased contact pressures across the joint articular surfaces, comparable to patho-biomechanical features following a total meniscectomy.[11] Root tears have been shown to be associated with high-grade chondral lesions, subchondral insufficiency fractures, progression of osteoarthritis, and increased joint instability.[12] Surgical repair with reattachment/fixation of posterior root tears is increasingly being performed arthroscopically, as nonoperative treatment has been associated with poor clinical outcomes.[13]

Successful surgical repair of meniscal root tears can be challenging, with techniques used including arthroscopic transtibial pullout repair (ATPR), suture anchor repair, and side-to-side repair.[14] Currently, the most commonly used technique for arthroscopic meniscal root repair is ATPR, in which anatomic repair of the torn meniscal root is facilitated using transosseous sutures through the proximal tibia.[10]

Meniscal Transplantation

In the setting of young and active patients with unicompartmental meniscal deficiency and a meniscal injury unamenable to repair, meniscal transplantation may be an option. Although meniscal transplants have been performed for more than 20 years, the procedure is still relatively uncommon and will not be covered in the context of the current review.

IMAGING TECHNIQUES
Conventional Magnetic Resonance Imaging

Protocols for conventional MR (cMR) imaging of the knee vary between institutions, but sequences usually comply with broadly accepted principles for detecting meniscal pathologic condition. Intermediate- and/or T1-weighted sequences, in both sagittal and coronal planes, are typically relied on to assess signal changes in the nonoperative meniscus.[15] However, a different approach is required after meniscal surgery. In this situation, an emphasis is placed on the acquisition and interpretation of T2-to-intermediate weighted fluid-sensitive acquisitions in sagittal and coronal planes to detect synovial fluid signal extending into the substance of the meniscus in the setting of a meniscal retear, indicating that the articular surface has been breached.

Direct Magnetic Resonance Arthrography

Direct MRA entails the intraarticular injection of 20 to 50 mL diluted gadolinium into the knee joint before MR examination.[16] Benefits of direct MRA include distention of the joint capsule, increased intraarticular pressure, reduced viscosity of the synovial fluid, and a high signal-to-noise ratio of diluted contrast on T1-weighted sequences.[17] The potential disadvantages of this technique compared with cMR imaging include radiation exposure if using fluoroscopic-guided injection techniques, small procedural risks such as infection, bleeding, allergic reaction, and physician time required to perform the injection as well as overall increased cost. For MRA, fat-saturated T1-weighted sequences are acquired in each of the principal anatomic planes, with a fat-saturated T2-weighted sequence performed in either the coronal or the sagittal plane to evaluate subchondral bone and exclude parameniscal cysts.[18]

Indirect Magnetic Resonance Arthrography

Indirect MRA is a less commonly used imaging alternative to direct MRA in the knee. Indirect MRA relies on the physiologic excretion and diffusion of intravascular gadolinium contrast into the joint through synovial cells of the joint capsule. Indirect MRA involves the intravenous administration of gadolinium-based contrast 20 to 90 minutes before MR imaging examination. Subsequently, patients are asked to exercise the knee before the MR imaging to promote synovial uptake and intraarticular diffusion of the contrast agent. The advantages of indirect MRA include its less-invasive means of introducing intraarticular contrast and its ability to identify sites of hyperemic synovitis or periarticular inflammation based on vascular tissue enhancement. As indirect MRA does not require direct joint injection, the contrast can be administered by a technologist rather than a physician. Shortcomings of this technique are increased patient time, increased costs and potential for adverse reactions to intravenous gadolinium contrast compared with cMR imaging, and lack of joint distention compared with direct MRA.[16] In addition, as some degree of enhancement in stable healed granulation tissue may be an expected finding in the postoperative meniscus and difficult to differentiate from a residual surfacing tear, indirect MRA may result in potential false positive findings in evaluation of recurrent or residual meniscal tearing.[8]

Computed Tomographic Arthrography

When MR imaging is contraindicated or unavailable, CTA may be performed to assess the postoperative meniscus. This technique entails the direct intraarticular administration of 20 to 50 mL diluted iodinated contrast agent into the knee joint. CTA examinations are acquired rapidly and with high-spatial resolution, and multiplanar reformatted images can be readily created from the initial data set. CT is unhindered by signal characteristics in the postoperative meniscus, as granulation tissue and intrasubstance degenerative signal.[16] CT and CTA imaging has superior spatial resolution when compared with MR imaging; however, the high-spatial resolution of CTA can lead to overinterpretation of subtle postoperative contour irregularities along margins of stable meniscal tissue, which may be inaccurately interpreted as indicative of residual/recurrent tearing.[19]

IMAGING FINDINGS
Meniscal Tears

A meniscal tear in a nonoperative knee is characterized on MR imaging by 2 main diagnostic criteria: either linear abnormal intrameniscal signal intensity on intermediate- or T1-weighted images extending into the superior or inferior surfaces of the meniscus, or the presence of altered normal meniscal morphology in the absence of prior surgery.[15] Using the "two-slice-touch" rule, which is defined as meniscal distortion or surfacing intrameniscal signal, seen on 2 or more consecutive slices, increases the likelihood of accurately diagnosing a meniscal tear on cMR imaging, as compared with observing such changes on only 1 MR image slice, with an increase in the positive predictive value from 91% to 94% for medial meniscal tears and from 83% to 96% for lateral meniscal tears.[20]

Postoperative Imaging

Before evaluating a postoperative meniscus, it is essential to recognize that surgery has been performed, particularly to avoid describing expected postoperative meniscal changes as indicative of a meniscal tear. Low-signal linear fibrotic stranding in Hoffa fat pad, focal thickening of the patellar tendon, and possible foci of magnetic susceptibility artifact from microscopic metallic fragments may be seen as MR imaging features of prior surgery.[21]

Imaging Findings after Meniscectomy

Partial resection of the meniscus is characterized by diminution of meniscal tissue, ranging from a large portion of the meniscus being removed to very mild blunting of the inner/apical margin of the meniscus (**Fig. 1**). Furthermore, mild irregularity of meniscal contour can be encountered, particularly in the first 6 to 9 months postoperatively, which tends to smooth out and remodel over time.[22] Such postoperative changes on MR imaging are particularly common following partial meniscectomy involving the posterior horn of the medial meniscus.

Following meniscectomy, intermediate-signal intensity extending to the articular surface of the postoperative meniscus on intermediate-weighted images may represent a tear, previous degenerative changes abutting the remnant meniscal neoarticular surface, or fibrovascular tissue in a healing tear.[23] This finding of surfacing signal on intermediate-weighted images was observed in 50% of arthroscopically proven untorn postoperative menisci in the study by White and colleagues,[24] and more than 50% of intact postoperative menisci in the study of Kijowski and colleagues.[22] Several investigations have similarly confirmed that intermediate-signal intensity extending into the articular surface on T2-

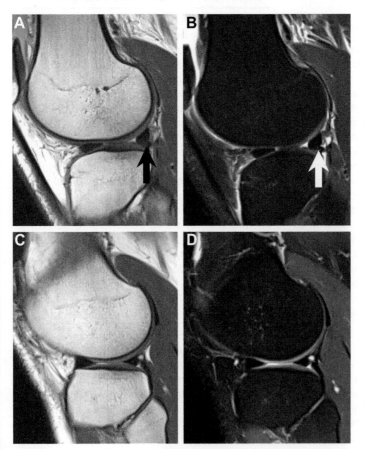

Fig. 1. A 19-year-old man before and following partial meniscectomy. Sagittal proton density (*A*) and sagittal fat-saturated T2-weighted images (*B*) showing a complex unstable tear of the posterior horn of the lateral meniscus. Blunting of the meniscal apex is present with an inferior and posteriorly flipped fragment (*arrow*). Sagittal proton density (*C*) and sagittal fat-saturated T2-weighted (*D*) images 2 years following partial meniscectomy show an intact and diminutive posterior horn of the lateral meniscus.

weighted images of a postoperative meniscus may be a nonspecific finding.[17,22,24–29] However, the absence of increased surfacing intrameniscal signal on intermediate- and T2-weighted imaging is a reliable negative predictive MR imaging finding of an intact postoperative meniscus.[22] The sensitivity of surfacing increased intrameniscal signal on intermediate-weighted and T2-weighted images in the diagnosis of a recurrent meniscal tear has been reported as 76% and 84%, respectively, by White and colleagues.[24] Lim and colleagues[27] found a sensitivity of 88% for surfacing intrameniscal signal on intermediate-weighted images. A recent study reported 100% sensitivity for surfacing intrameniscal increased intermediate- and T2-weighted signal in the diagnosis of a torn postoperative meniscus.[22] The specificity of surfacing fluidlike intrameniscal T2 signal for the detection of a torn postoperative meniscus has been reported between 88% and 90%.[17,27] A recent study found that surfacing intrameniscal intermediate- to high-signal or high signal in a postoperative meniscus on T2-weighted MR images was a reliable finding of a meniscal retear with a specificity of 96% (**Fig. 2**). An important diagnostic consideration following partial meniscectomy is that horizontal tears, unlike other types of meniscal tears, do not have to be completely excised, and a horizontal cleft, extending into the articular surface, may be present in the setting of a stable residual meniscus after partial meniscectomy and may be misinterpreted as a recurrent or residual meniscal tear.[18]

In the scenario whereby an MR imaging examination of the knee before meniscectomy is available for comparison, the finding of new areas of increased intrameniscal surfacing T2 signal on postoperative MR imaging has been described as resulting in diagnostic sensitivity of 86% and specificity of 98% in the diagnosis of a recurrent

meniscal tear.[22] This emphasizes the importance and clinical value of comparing MR imaging findings postoperatively to baseline preoperative examinations whenever possible.

The diagnostic performance of postoperative MR imaging following prior partial meniscectomy has been shown to be dependent on the amount of meniscal tissue resected. Studies have shown that cMR imaging has a diagnostic accuracy as high as 89% to 100% for meniscal retears in the setting of meniscectomy less than 25%, but performs less adequately with diagnostic accuracy dropping to 65% to 78% when greater than 25% of meniscal tissue has been resected.[17,24]

Based on these findings and inherent limitations of cMR imaging, MRA has been advocated as an alternative diagnostic technique in the assessment of patients with greater than 25% meniscectomy. Similar to prior investigators, Magee and colleagues[30] reported that cMR imaging was accurate for the diagnosis of a recurrent or residual meniscal tear in all patients with prior meniscectomy involving less than 25% of the meniscus; however, MRA was necessary to accurately diagnose a meniscal retear in 26% of patients. The advantage of direct MRA lies in its ability to highlight a meniscus retear owing to imbibition of contrast agent into the torn segment, which should appear isointense to gadolinium in joint fluid on T1-weighted images (**Fig. 3**). However, not all meniscus retears show this finding.[28,31] The absence of intrameniscal extension of contrast into a site of tearing is possibly due to partial volume averaging, mechanical obstruction to uptake in slitlike tears, or granulation tissue at the neoarticular outer margin.[16]

The diagnostic accuracy in the detection of a recurrent tear after partial meniscectomy was reported to range from 57% to 80% for cMR imaging, 85% to 93% for direct MRA, and 81% to

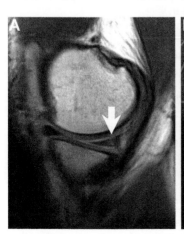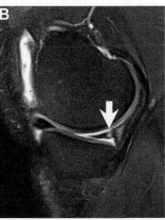

Fig. 2. A 31-year-old man with prior partial meniscectomy. Recurrent peripheral tear in the posterior horn of the medial meniscus with surfacing intermediate signal on sagittal proton density acquisitions (*A*) and intermediate- to high-intrameniscal signal extending to the meniscal articular surface (*arrows*) on sagittal fat-saturated T2-weighted images (*B*).

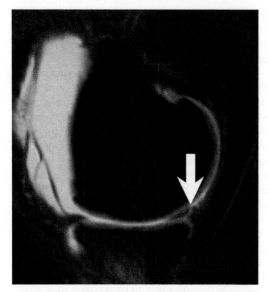

Fig. 3. A 35-year-old woman with recurrent tear following prior partial meniscectomy. MRA shows a recurrent vertical longitudinal tear in the posterior horn of the medial meniscus (*arrow*). The retear is highlighted because of imbibition of contrast agent into the torn segment, appearing isointense to gadolinium in joint fluid on T1-weighted fat-suppressed images.

93% for indirect MRA.[17,24,25,27,29,32] For direct and indirect MRA, increased sensitivity and specificity for the diagnosis of meniscus retear generally have been noted, compared with cMR imaging. However, a randomized cohort study comparing the performance of cMR imaging, MRA, and indirect MRA found no statistical difference among the 3 techniques for the diagnosis of a recurrent meniscal tear, although there was a trend toward increased sensitivity, specificity, and accuracy for both direct and indirect MRA compared with cMR imaging.[24]

Most studies evaluating residual or recurrent meniscal tears have been performed using field strengths of 1.5 T or less. One study, however, evaluated 3-T cMR imaging versus direct MRA.[28] Results of this investigation showed that at 3-T imaging MRA had a higher sensitivity than cMR imaging (88% compared with 78%) and higher specificity (100% and 85%). The study did not include a comparison with a 1.5-T field strength imaging.

CTA has been compared with second-look arthroscopy in a retrospective study following partial meniscectomy.[19] Criteria for recurrent tearing included contrast imbibition in the postoperative meniscus, separation of the meniscus from the capsule, or visualization of a displaced meniscal fragment. Retrospective interpretation of CTA

examinations with the use of these criteria yielded a sensitivity of 93% and a specificity of 89% in the CTA diagnosis of a meniscal retear (**Fig. 4**).

Imaging Findings after Meniscal Repair

In the repaired meniscus, intrinsic high signal may be seen within the meniscus related to healing with early fibrovascular response and the subsequent development of a fibrocartilaginous scar.[24,33,34] This results in MR imaging features of mildly increased intermediate and T2 signal along healing and healed meniscal repair sites again mimicking the features of a preoperative meniscal tear. In studies of meniscal repair, Farley and colleagues[26] found surfacing increased signal on short TE images in more than 60% of intact meniscal repairs. Similar results were demonstrated by Miao and colleagues,[35] with approximately half of the patients with intact menisci illustrating features of surfacing increased intermediate-weighted linear signal at the healed repair site (**Fig. 5**). The specificity of cMR imaging for the detection of a residual or recurrent tear has been shown to improve using diagnostic criteria of T2-weighted fluidlike signal extending into a meniscal repair interface, albeit with relatively low sensitivity (**Figs. 6** and **7**).[26,36,37] Diastasis of the edges of the meniscal repair by more than 1 mm has been demonstrated to be a useful, but infrequent sign in the diagnosis of recurrent tears following prior meniscal repair (**Fig. 8**).[38]

On MRA, in general, 2 patterns of intrameniscal contrast imbibition can be seen in the setting of a failed or retorn meniscal repair. The first pattern is the extension of intraarticular contrast through the meniscal repair site from 1 articular surface to another, as may occur in the setting of a failed repair or a full-thickness recurrent tear. The second pattern is the extension of intraarticular contrast into a portion of the meniscus and may represent a partially healed repair or a partial thickness recurrent tear.[18]

The reported accuracy for diagnosing a residual of recurrent tear after meniscal repair in the literature has ranged from 57% to 80% for cMR imaging, from 85% to 93% for direct MRA, and from 81% to 93% for indirect MRA. Several studies concluded that direct MRA is superior to cMR imaging,[17,25,29,30,32] with other studies showing diagnostic equivalence between direct MRA and indirect MRA in the detection of recurrent or residual meniscal tearing in patients after meniscus repair.[24,32]

Imaging Findings After Meniscal Root Repair

Following meniscal root repair, MR imaging can be valuable in the evaluation of meniscus position, the

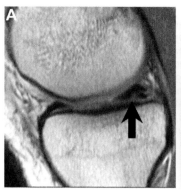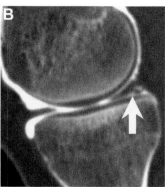

Fig. 4. A 47-year-old man with recurrent meniscal tear following prior meniscal repair. Recurrent tear of the posterior horn of the medial meniscus with surfacing intermediate signal (*black arrow*) on proton density images (*A*) and corresponding CTA showing contrast imbibition (*white arrow*) in the meniscal retear (*B*).

healing status of the fixed meniscal root, and the tunnel position after ATPR.[39] MR imaging features of successful meniscal root repair and healing have been described, including maintained reduction of the medial meniscus posterior root to its anatomic attachment, continuity of meniscal root insertion to the tibia in all 3 planes, normal low or intermediate-signal intensity of the root repair insertion site on T1-weighted imaging, and no

disruption or discontinuity of the meniscal root insertion on T2-weighted imaging (**Fig. 9**). Partial healing has been described as loss of visualized continuity of the root insertion in 1 plane and nonhealing as loss of continuity in all planes on MR imaging.[40–42]

The anatomic position of the posterior root insertion of the posterior horn medial meniscus is typically 5 to 8 mm anteromedial to the most

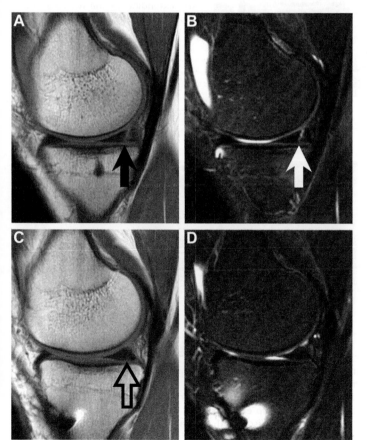

Fig. 5. A 23-year-old man, preoperative and postoperative imaging following successful meniscal repair. Sagittal proton density (*A*) and sagittal fat-saturated T2-weighted images (*B*) show a vertical longitudinal tear of the posterior horn of the medial meniscus. Sagittal proton density (*C*) and sagittal fat-saturated T2-weighted images (*D*) 1 year postmeniscal repair show an intact repair with mildly increased surfacing signal on proton density imaging (*open black arrow* in *C*).

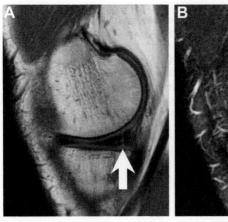
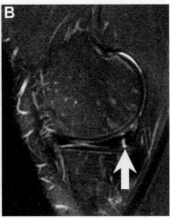

Fig. 6. A 30-year-old man with recurrent tear following prior meniscal repair. Recurrent vertical longitudinal tear in the posterior horn of the medial meniscus with surfacing increased signal on sagittal proton density (A) and fluidlike signal on corresponding fat-suppressed T2-weighted imaging (B) extending to the meniscal articular surface (arrows).

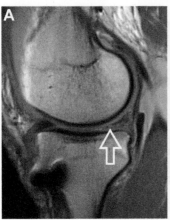
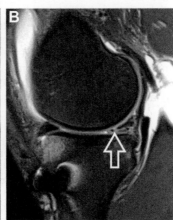

Fig. 7. A 29-year old woman. Recurrent meniscal tear, 1 year postmeniscal repair and ACL reconstruction. Recurrent/residual complex tear of the posterior horn of the medial meniscus with surfacing increased signal on sagittal proton density (A) and fluidlike signal on corresponding fat-suppressed T2-weighted imaging (B), extending to the meniscal articular surface (arrows).

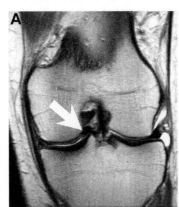
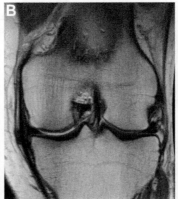
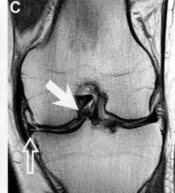

Fig. 8. A 38-year-old woman. Recurrent bucket-handle tear following medial meniscus repair. Coronal intermediate-weighted images (A–C). Preoperative examination shows a large centrally displaced bucket-handle tear of the medial meniscus (arrow in A). Imaging 1 year postrepair (B), the medial meniscus appears intact with no increased surfacing meniscal signal. Follow-up examination 4 years after initial repair (C) shows a recurrent displaced bucket-handle tear of the medial meniscus with centrally displaced meniscal tissue again noted in the intercondylar notch (arrow) and peripheral extrusion of the residual component of the body medial meniscus (open arrow).

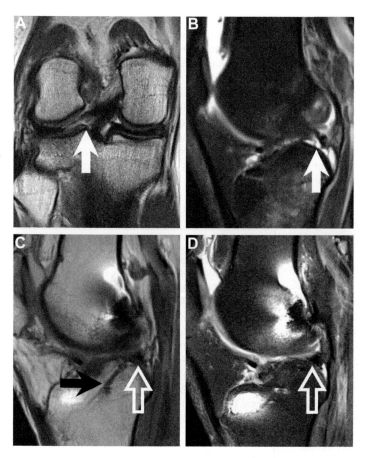

Fig. 9. A 26-year-old woman before and following posterior root repair, lateral meniscus. Coronal proton density (*A*) and sagittal fat-saturated T2-weighted (*B*) images show a complete tear of the posterior root insertion of the lateral meniscus (*arrows*). Sagittal proton density (*C*) and fat-saturated T2-weighted (*D*) images 2 years following posterior root repair show an intact root insertion (*open white arrows*) with fixation suture tract through the proximal tibia (*black arrow in C*).

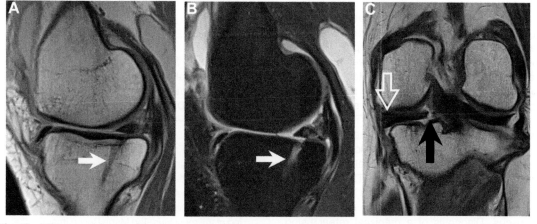

Fig. 10. A 33-year-old man with recurrent tear following prior posterior medial meniscus root repair. Sagittal proton density (*A*), sagittal fat-saturated T2-weighted (*B*) and coronal intermediate-weighted (*C*) images illustrate increased signal and discontinuity of the posterior root of the medial meniscus. Transosseous fixation suture tracks (*white arrows*) can be seen in the tibia extending to the site of the posterior root repair. A full-thickness recurrent radial tear seen of the posterior horn medial meniscus at its posterior root insertion (*black arrow*), with associated secondary peripheral extrusion of the medial meniscus from the joint line (*open arrow*).

superior tibial attachment of the posterior cruciate ligament.[43] Hiranaka and colleagues[44] showed that following ATPR the distance between the root repair tibial suture tunnel aperture and the anticipated anatomic meniscal root attachment site was correlated with meniscal root healing, with anatomic repair within 5.8 mm of the anticipated root insertion site associated with better healing outcomes. MR imaging criteria for a repeat or new tear after ATPR include increased signal intensity extending through the root attachment to the articular surface on T2-weighted images correlating to loss of tissue continuity at the meniscal root repair site, displaced meniscal root fragments, or abnormal surfacing intrameniscal signal at a site distant from the root repair site (**Fig. 10**).[14]

Important Considerations for the Day-to-Day Practice

When evaluating patients after meniscal surgery, it should be considered that the status of the meniscus is not the only clinical question in many cases. Joint-line pain after meniscal surgery may result from either recurrent or residual meniscal abnormalities or other causes, such as acute traumatic cartilage lesions, local osteoarthritis, and changes in the subchondral marrow of the femur or tibia, including insufficiency fractures or other derangement of the joint. The imaging modality selected in evaluation of patients following meniscal surgery should be robust enough to evaluate the meniscus as well as the cartilage, bone, and surrounding soft tissues.

SUMMARY

Meniscal tearing is among the most common knee pathologic conditions. Surgical treatment options in the setting of an unstable meniscal tear are partial meniscectomy and meniscal repair. Posterior meniscus root repairs involve newer techniques developed to reestablish and maintain stability of root insertions of the menisci. The primary goals and principles of modern meniscal surgery are to reestablish stability in the residual meniscus and to preserve as much meniscal tissue as possible.

Standard MR imaging diagnostic criteria of a meniscal tear, including abnormal morphology and surfacing intrameniscal short TE signal, may be normal postoperative findings complicating the MR imaging assessment of the postoperative meniscus. Diagnosis of a meniscal retear using cMR imaging, MRA, or CTA is primarily dependent on imaging features of fluid imbibition into a residual or recurrent cleft within the meniscal substance, nonsurgical morphologic abnormalities, including fragmentation or anatomic discontinuity,

or visualization of a displaced meniscal fragment. Prior investigations have demonstrated that MRA may have an improved accuracy over cMR imaging particularly when there has been a prior meniscectomy greater than 25%. However, in cases with prior meniscectomy less than 25%, the accuracy between cMR imaging and direct MRA has been shown to be equivalent. CTA is the recommended alternative for patients who are unable to undergo MR examination or for cases in which extensive artifact from implants obscures the meniscus.

CLINICS CARE POINTS

- MR imaging performed without or with intraarticular contrast agent is the examination of choice for assessing patients who have recurrent symptoms after meniscus surgery.

- The evaluation of the postoperative meniscus with MR imaging can be challenging, as standard MR diagnostic criteria of a meniscal tear may be normal findings postoperatively.

- When evaluating a postoperative meniscus, the diagnosis of a recurrent or residual meniscal tear is primarily based on the visualization of surfacing high intrameniscal T2-weighted "fluid" signal, or intrameniscal contrast material on MR or computed tomographic arthrography.

DISCLOSURE

The authors have nothing to disclose.

REFERENCES

1. Montgomery SR, Zhang A, Ngo SS, et al. Cross-sectional analysis of trends in meniscectomy and meniscus repair. Orthopedics 2013;36(8):e1007–13.
2. McDermott ID, Amis AA. The consequences of meniscectomy. J Bone Joint Surg Br 2006;88(12):1549–56.
3. Boutin RD, Fritz RC, Marder RA. Magnetic resonance imaging of the postoperative meniscus: resection, repair, and replacement. Magn Reson Imaging Clin N Am 2014;22(4):517–55.
4. Rosas HG, De Smet AA. Magnetic resonance imaging of the meniscus. Top Magn Reson Imaging 2009;20(3):151–73.
5. Robson MD, Gatehouse PD, Bydder M, et al. Magnetic resonance: an introduction to ultrashort TE (UTE) imaging. J Comput Assist Tomogr 2003;27(6):825–46.

6. Nguyen JC, De Smet AA, Graf BK, et al. MR imaging-based diagnosis and classification of meniscal tears. Radiographics 2014;34(4):981–99.

7. Starke C, Kopf S, Petersen W, et al. Meniscal repair. Arthroscopy 2009;25(9):1033–44.

8. Sanders TG. Imaging of the postoperative knee. Semin Musculoskelet Radiol 2011;15(4):383–407.

9. Fox MG. MR imaging of the meniscus: review, current trends, and clinical implications. Radiol Clin North Am 2007;45(6):1033–53, vii.

10. Feucht MJ, Izadpanah K, Lacheta L, et al. Arthroscopic transtibial pullout repair for posterior meniscus root tears. Oper Orthop Traumatol 2019;31(3):248–60.

11. Feucht MJ, Kuhle J, Bode G, et al. Arthroscopic transtibial pullout repair for posterior medial meniscus root tears: a systematic review of clinical, radiographic, and second-look arthroscopic results. Arthroscopy 2015;31(9):1808–16.

12. Guermazi A, Hayashi D, Jarraya M, et al. Medial posterior meniscal root tears are associated with development or worsening of medial tibiofemoral cartilage damage: the multicenter osteoarthritis study. Radiology 2013;268(3):814–21.

13. Kamatsuki Y, Furumatsu T, Miyazawa S, et al. The early arthroscopic pullout repair of medial meniscus posterior root tear is more effective for reducing medial meniscus extrusion. Acta Med Okayama 2019;73(6):503–10.

14. Palisch AR, Winters RR, Willis MH, et al. Posterior root meniscal tears: preoperative, intraoperative, and postoperative imaging for transtibial pullout repair. Radiographics 2016;36(6):1792–806.

15. De Smet AA, Norris MA, Yandow DR, et al. MR diagnosis of meniscal tears of the knee: importance of high signal in the meniscus that extends to the surface. AJR Am J Roentgenol 1993; 161(1):101–7.

16. Baker JC, Friedman MV, Rubin DA. Imaging the postoperative knee meniscus: an evidence-based review. AJR Am J Roentgenol 2018;211(3):519–27.

17. Applegate GR, Flannigan BD, Tolin BS, et al. MR diagnosis of recurrent tears in the knee: value of intraarticular contrast material. AJR Am J Roentgenol 1993;161(4):821–5.

18. Toms AP, White LM, Marshall TJ, et al. Imaging the post-operative meniscus. Eur J Radiol 2005;54(2): 189–98.

19. Mutschler C, Vande Berg BC, Lecouvet FE, et al. Postoperative meniscus: assessment at dual-detector row spiral CT arthrography of the knee. Radiology 2003;228(3):635–41.

20. De Smet AA. How I diagnose meniscal tears on knee MRI. AJR Am J Roentgenol 2012;199(3): 481–99.

21. Morrison W, Sanders T. Imaging of the knee. In: Problem solving in musculoskeletal Imaging. Philadelphia: Mosby/Elsevier; 2008. p. 634.

22. Kijowski R, Rosas H, Williams A, et al. MRI characteristics of torn and untorn post-operative menisci. Skeletal Radiol 2017;46(10):1353–60.

23. McCauley TR. MR imaging evaluation of the postoperative knee. Radiology 2005;234(1):53–61.

24. White LM, Schweitzer ME, Weishaupt D, et al. Diagnosis of recurrent meniscal tears: prospective evaluation of conventional MR imaging, indirect MR arthrography, and direct MR arthrography. Radiology 2002;222(2):421–9.

25. Ciliz D, Ciliz A, Elverici E, et al. Evaluation of postoperative menisci with MR arthrography and routine conventional MRI. Clin Imaging 2008;32(3):212–9.

26. Farley TE, Howell SM, Love KF, et al. Meniscal tears: MR and arthrographic findings after arthroscopic repair. Radiology 1991;180(2):517–22.

27. Lim PS, Schweitzer ME, Bhatia M, et al. Repeat tear of postoperative meniscus: potential MR imaging signs. Radiology 1999;210(1):183–8.

28. Magee T. Accuracy of 3-Tesla MR and MR arthrography in diagnosis of meniscal retear in the postoperative knee. Skeletal Radiol 2014;43(8):1057–64.

29. Sciulli RL, Boutin RD, Brown RR, et al. Evaluation of the postoperative meniscus of the knee: a study comparing conventional arthrography, conventional MR imaging, MR arthrography with iodinated contrast material, and MR arthrography with gadolinium-based contrast material. Skeletal Radiol 1999;28(9):508–14.

30. Magee T, Shapiro M, Rodriguez J, et al. MR arthrography of postoperative knee: for which patients is it useful? Radiology 2003;229(1):159–63.

31. De Smet AA, Horak DM, Davis KW, et al. Intensity of signal contacting meniscal surface in recurrent tears on MR arthrography compared with that of contrast material. AJR Am J Roentgenol 2006;187(6): W565–8.

32. Vives MJ, Homesley D, Ciccotti MG, et al. Evaluation of recurring meniscal tears with gadolinium-enhanced magnetic resonance imaging: a randomized, prospective study. Am J Sports Med 2003;31(6):868–73.

33. Deutsch AL, Mink JH, Fox JM, et al. Peripheral meniscal tears: MR findings after conservative treatment or arthroscopic repair. Radiology 1990;176(2):485–8.

34. Viala P, Marchand P, Lecouvet F, et al. Imaging of the postoperative knee. Diagn Interv Imaging 2016; 97(7–8):823–37.

35. Miao Y, Yu JK, Ao YF, et al. Diagnostic values of 3 methods for evaluating meniscal healing status after meniscal repair: comparison among second-look arthroscopy, clinical assessment, and magnetic resonance imaging. Am J Sports Med 2011;39(4): 735–42.

36. Mariani PP, Santori N, Adriani E, et al. Accelerated rehabilitation after arthroscopic meniscal repair: a clinical and magnetic resonance imaging evaluation. Arthroscopy 1996;12(6):680–6.

37. Trattnig S, Rand T, Czerny C, et al. Magnetic resonance imaging of the postoperative knee. Top Magn Reson Imaging 1999;10(4):221–36.

38. Recht MP, Kramer J. MR imaging of the postoperative knee: a pictorial essay. Radiographics 2002; 22(4):765–74.

39. Okazaki Y, Furumatsu T, Masuda S, et al. Pullout repair of the medial meniscus posterior root tear reduces proton density-weighted imaging signal intensity of the medial meniscus. Acta Med Okayama 2018;72(5):493–8.

40. Kim JH, Chung JH, Lee DH, et al. Arthroscopic suture anchor repair versus pullout suture repair in posterior root tear of the medial meniscus: a prospective comparison study. Arthroscopy 2011; 27(12):1644–53.

41. Kim SB, Ha JK, Lee SW, et al. Medial meniscus root tear refixation: comparison of clinical, radiologic, and arthroscopic findings with medial meniscectomy. Arthroscopy 2011;27(3):346–54.

42. Moon HK, Koh YG, Kim YC, et al. Prognostic factors of arthroscopic pull-out repair for a posterior root tear of the medial meniscus. Am J Sports Med 2012;40(5):1138–43.

43. Johannsen AM, Civitarese DM, Padalecki JR, et al. Qualitative and quantitative anatomic analysis of the posterior root attachments of the medial and lateral menisci. Am J Sports Med 2012;40(10): 2342–7.

44. Hiranaka T, Furumatsu T, Kamatsuki Y, et al. The distance between the tibial tunnel aperture and meniscal root attachment is correlated with meniscal healing status following transtibial pullout repair for medial meniscus posterior root tear. Knee 2020; 27(3):899–905.

Moving?

Make sure your subscription moves with you!

To notify us of your new address, find your **Clinics Account Number** (located on your mailing label above your name), and contact customer service at:

Email: journalscustomerservice-usa@elsevier.com

800-654-2452 (subscribers in the U.S. & Canada)
314-447-8871 (subscribers outside of the U.S. & Canada)

Fax number: 314-447-8029

Elsevier Health Sciences Division
Subscription Customer Service
3251 Riverport Lane
Maryland Heights, MO 63043

*To ensure uninterrupted delivery of your subscription, please notify us at least 4 weeks in advance of move.

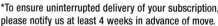

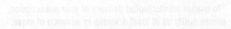

Printed and bound by CPI Group (UK) Ltd, Croydon, CR0 4YY

08/05/2025

01864700-0014

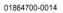